Pocket Guide to Teaching for Medical Instructors

D0715418

Pocket Guide to Teaching for Medical Instructors

Second Edition

Advanced Life Support Group and
Resuscitation Council (UK)

Edited by
**Ian Bullock, Mike Davis, Andrew Lockey
and Kevin Mackway-Jones**

Blackwell
Publishing

BMJ|Books

© 1998 by BMJ Books
© 2008 by Blackwell Publishing
BMJ Books is an imprint of the BMJ Publishing Group Limited, used under licence

Blackwell Publishing, Inc., 350 Main Street, Malden, Massachusetts 02148-5020, USA
Blackwell Publishing Ltd, 9600 Garsington Road, Oxford OX4 2DQ, UK
Blackwell Publishing Asia Pty Ltd, 550 Swanston Street, Carlton, Victoria 3053, Australia

First published 1998 by BMJ
Second Edition 2008

1   2008

Library of Congress Cataloging-in-Publication Data

Pocket guide to teaching for medical instructors / Advanced Life Support
Group and Resuscitation Council (UK); edited by Ian Bullock ... [et al.]. -- 2nd ed.
    p. ; cm.
    Rev. ed. of: The pocket guide to teaching for medical instructors / Advanced Life Support Group; edited
by Kevin Mackway-Jones and Mike Walker in collaboration with the Resuscitation Council (UK). 1998.
    Includes bibliographical references and index.
    ISBN 978-1-4051-7569-2 (alk. paper)
    1. Medical teaching personnel--Training of. 2. Teaching--Methodology. 3. Learning strategies.
I. Bullock, Ian. II. Advanced Life Support Group (Manchester, England)
    [DNLM: 1. Teaching--methods. 2. Health Personnel--education. W 18 P739 2008]

    R833.5.P63 2008
    610.71'1--dc22
                                                                                    2007047281
ISBN: 978-1-4051-7569-2

A catalogue record for this title is available from the British Library

Set in 9.25/12 pt Meridien by Charon Tec Ltd (A Macmillan Company), Chennai, India
www.charontec.com

Printed and bound in Singapore by Utopia Press Pte Ltd

Commissioning Editor: Mary Banks
Development Editor: Simone Dudziak
Production Controller: Rachel Edwards

For further information on Blackwell Publishing, visit our Website:
http://www.blackwellpublishing.com

Contents

Working group

Kathy Boardman
Manchester

Ian Bullock
Oxford

Mike Davis
Blackpool

Andrew Lockey
Halifax

Kevin Mackway-Jones
Manchester

Sarah Mitchell
London

Sean Russell
London

Sue Wieteska
Manchester

Contributors to the Second Edition

Ian Bullock
Oxford

Mike Davis
Blackpool

Kate Denning
Plymouth

Peter Driscoll
Manchester

Carl Gwinnutt
Manchester

Andrew Lockey
Halifax

Kevin Mackie
Birmingham

Kevin Mackway-Jones
Manchester

Sarah Mitchell
London

Gavin Perkins
Birmingham

Russell Perkins
Manchester

Sue Wieteska
Manchester

Jonathan Wyllie
Middlesbrough

Jackie Younker
Bristol

Contributors to the First Edition of the *Pocket Guide to Teaching for Medical Instructors* and/or *ALS Instructor Manual*

Ian Bullock
Oxford

Andrew Coleman
Northampton

Mick Colquhoun
Cardiff

Pat Conaghan
Manchester

Mike Davis
Blackpool

Peter Driscoll
Manchester

David Gabbott
Bristol

Carl Gwinnutt
Manchester

Bob Harris
London

Duncan Harris
London

Sara Harris
London

Jane Hatfield
Oxford

Gareth Holsgrove
Cambridge

Pauline Howard
Oxford

Melanie Humphreys
Wolverhampton

Lynn Jones
Manchester

Andrew Lockey
Halifax

Kevin Mackway-Jones
Manchester

Sarah Mitchell
London

Jerry Nolan
Oxford

Gavin Perkins
Birmingham

Mike Walker
London

Terence Wardle
Chester

Celia Warlow
Northampton

Sue Wieteska
Manchester

Preface to the Second Edition

This, the second edition of the 'Blue Book', has quite an act to follow. For the past ten years potential instructors around the world have enjoyed receiving and reading the Pocket Guide – both as a symbol of their progression to instructor status, and also as a valuable resource to aid their teaching practice.

The time is now right to update the guide with best current educational practice and to also incorporate some of the suggestions and changes that had been made by the thousands of instructors who have used it. This edition sticks to the underlying principle of the first – to provide a pocket sized guide to the basics of good instructor practice. A number of new concepts, above and beyond those previously used, have been incorporated. Current instructors will particularly appreciate the updating of the adult learning section, the clarity of the revised 'active' chapters and the incorporation of key references and further reading that will allow those who wish to, to deepen understanding of the subject. To reflect current trends a completely new chapter on e-learning has also been included.

Everyone who has the pleasure of instructing knows what a privilege it can be to share knowledge with motivated students. It is even more enjoyable if the teaching is done so well that the unmotivated and less able are fully engaged. We cannot guarantee your success following the reading of this little book, but we can at least say that the beginning of your journey to becoming a good teacher will be based on firm foundations after doing so. You will probably come back to the principles espoused here again and again as you reflect on what does and doesn't work for you. We echo our original exhortation of ten years ago:

Good luck, and enjoy your teaching.

Ian Bullock
Mike Davis
Andrew Lockey
Kevin Mackway-Jones
(Editorial Board)

Preface to the First Edition

This short guide is in two parts. Part one begins by introducing the basic principles under teaching and then goes on to deal in more detail with a number of modes of teaching on courses. Lectures skill stations, scenarios, workshops and discussions are dealt with here. In each case practical guidance is given to help the reader to become a more effective teacher.

Part two covers many of the same areas again, but this time giving more background information, and describing some more advanced instructional skills. It deals with the nature of adult learning, the four domains of learning, the learning process, questions and answers, role play, mentoring and problems with workshops and discussions. Each topic is presented as a short section which can be sampled to help with specific issues.

The guide is intended as an aid to reflection: something which you can, and hopefully will, consult on many occasions before, during and after your courses. It does not contain all the answers, but it will at least provide an alternative voice, something to argue with and something against which you can test your experiences. This guide does not attempt to provide a blueprint for teaching, rather it gives advice about the basics which, once mastered will be adapted to your personality and creativity. In the end, of course, it is what works for you that matters.

In the long run it does not matter greatly whether you read this guide before or after a course (although most courses will require you to read beforehand). Knowledge and skill as a teacher build up gradually, provided you are able to reflect upon your teaching experiences and continue to learn.

Good luck with your teaching.

Mike Walker
Kevin Mackway-Jones
(Editorial Board)

Acknowledgments

A great many people have put a lot of hard work into the production of this book, and the accompanying generic instructor course. The editors would like to thank all the contributors for their efforts.

Finally, we would like to thank, in advance, those of you who will attend the Generic Instructor Course; no doubt, you will have much constructive criticism to offer.

CHAPTER 1
Adult learning

Learning outcomes

By the end of this chapter you should be able to demonstrate an understanding of:
• How adults learn
• An experiential learning cycle
• How best to improve motivation

Introduction

While adult learners differ from children and adolescents in a wide variety of ways (largely as a consequence of the voluntary character of adult learning), they retain some characteristics, particularly a perceived need to see the teacher as a repository of knowledge and insight. In general, however, adult learners (and health professionals in particular) can be thought of as having the capacity to demonstrate different attributes (Knowles, 1973).

Autonomy and self-determination

These are not always possible in formal learning but in general, health professionals have at least the capacity to take decisions about the direction and timing of their learning. Where decisions are taken out of their hands – for example by being sent on a course – there may be some initial resistance unless learning can be experienced as stimulating and valuable.

Pocket Guide to Teaching for Medical Instructors, Second Edition. Edited by Ian Bullock, Mike Davis, Andrew Lockey and Kevin Mackway-Jones. © 2008 Blackwell Publishing, ISBN: 978-1-4051-7569-2.

Life experience and knowledge

Most health professionals have had many years of formal full-time education (13 years in school, 3–6 years in university) and many years more in postgraduate training. No matter how receptive they may be to new ideas, there is a great deal of conservatism which needs to be overcome before learning can occur. This has been represented by Lewin (1951) in the following way:

Unfreezing → change → refreezing

Unfreezing is the point at which the learner becomes open to the idea of change (in understanding, affect, skill level); change is then incorporated and reinforced through feedback (see Chapter 8).

Goal orientated

Many adults like to have an outcome or a clear product from their efforts. Learning for its own sake may have some attractions at certain times, but it is not a luxury that busy professionals can include in their working lives.

Relevance orientated

Similarly, learning has to be relevant to work-based practices if it is to be valued by learners. As well as subject matter, this also relates to level: material can fail to be relevant if it is too easy or too complex. Content needs to be constructed around the experiences of the learner.

Practical

Learners get a great deal from integrating skills, knowledge and affect in complex, practical learning events, preferably related to previous experience and/or expectation of future practice. As a recent candidate on a European Provider Course wrote:

... we are not machines and this course gives room for us to think and makes the whole teaching session and the teamwork alive and interesting. It opens up for discussions and that is where you really learn something – not only from the instructors but also from the other candidates.

(Nana Gitz Holler, Denmark)

Esteem

Ask health professionals about negative experiences of learning and they are likely to mention humiliation. Good education acknowledges the contribution that learners can make to the

learning of others including the teachers (and respects their achieve-
ments thus far).

The experiential learning cycle

There are a number of theories of adult learning that are relevant to those involved in continuing medical education, but it is
beyond the scope of this book to explore them all. Relevant titles
are included in Chapter 11 for those who are interested in exploring some of these. However, there is one theory that is useful to
explore briefly here, that of experiential learning.

This theory was based on ideas about reflection developed in the
1930s by John Dewey (1938). One of the components is the experiential learning cycle, illustrated in Figure 1.1.

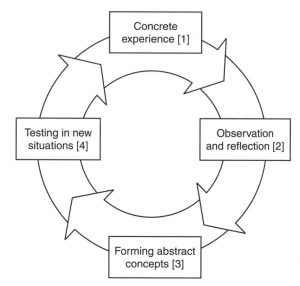

Figure 1.1 Experiential learning cycle.

This model, attributed to Kolb and Fry (1975), is a helpful source
of explanation for what we do all the time. We have hundreds of
experiences every day but most of them pass us by. If, however,
we are to learn from them, we have to be willing and able to go
round the cycle.

Experience, any event, however small. Enabling learners to utilise
experience provides the foundation for them to maximise learning.

Observation and reflection is the process of describing the event and trying to understand its significance. This stage can sometimes be captured by asking the following questions:
• What happened?
• What did it feel like?
These questions are intended to enable the learner to look in some detail at events and identify some of their emotional components.

Forming abstract concepts is an attempt to generalise from the specific, by asking:
• What does it mean?
• Do I need to change?
Take as an example, being late for a workshop. The focus of your observation and reflection will (inevitably) be related to that specific event, that is being late on that occasion and your thinking might be: '*The next time I am due to lead a workshop, I will set off a little earlier*'. The conceptualisation phase, however, will explore being late in other contexts and the generalisation would be framed in more general terms, thus: '*When I am due to go somewhere to do something, I will set off earlier than I think I need to, just in case something holds me up on the way*'. This kind of thinking, therefore leads into:

Testing in new situations, considering the question:
• How might I be different in the future?
Note that it is '*I*' being different. It is easier to change your own behaviour than it is to change that of others.

By going round the experiential learning cycle, a learner can capitalise on personal insight into events that are often taken for granted, but which can benefit from closer examination. Most experiences probably do not justify this exploration, but if behaviour seems to be working against us (e.g. as in the case of being habitually late), there is some real merit in exploring experience in a more systematic way.

In the context of continuing medical education, the experiential learning cycle has the merit of the systematic, shared exploration of repeat practice in a controlled environment, with feedback and discussion seeking to achieve improvement and develop competence which can be employed back in the workplace (see Chapter 8).

Maximising motivation

Adult learners have to be motivated if they are going to learn and the principle of voluntarism is a key feature of successful adult learning experiences. Almost by definition, learners in continual medical education contexts will be voluntary – in that nobody is forcing them to attend a programme. Nevertheless, they may be extrinsically motivated, that is the factors that are influencing their attendance may be driven by outside forces. In the context of continuing medical education these include gaining recognition, having something to put on a CV, or filling a need for career progression.

Malone and Lepper (1987) has detailed how intrinsic motivation has different, and predominantly internal, drivers and these can be summarised as in Table 1.1.

Table 1.1 Intrinsic motivation

Factors	Elements
Challenge	Meaningful goals that challenge learners just beyond their comfort zones
Curiosity	An expectation that there may be better ways of doing things; that there are things that you do not know
Independence	Learners demonstrating the need to move towards autonomy
Imagination	The capacity to work in 'let's pretend' environments (see particularly Chapter 5) where risks can be taken in safety
Social comparison	The desire to judge personal performance against that of others
Interdependence	The willingness to contribute towards others' learning
Esteem	Knowing that success will contribute towards feeling good about oneself

Extrinsic motivation is often regarded as 'bad' in comparison to 'good' intrinsic motivation, and it is generally true that people are more likely to own up to intrinsic drivers when asked, for example, why they are attending a course. It is likely that most individuals are motivated both extrinsically and intrinsically. Those motivated solely by external factors can, however, still be effective learners if certain needs are met.

Most reports of Maslow's hierarchy of needs (1971) have five layers in the pyramid but the model shown in Figure 1.2 acknowledges his later thinking.

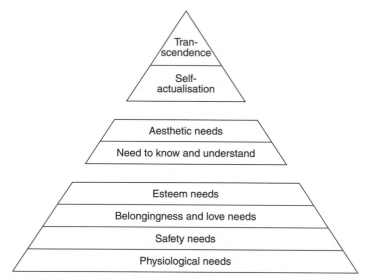

Figure 1.2 Maslow's hierarchy of needs (http://chiron.valdosta.edu/whuitt/ COL/motivation/motivate.html).

This classical theory of motivation demands that much of the lower-level needs have to be met before the learner can move up to the next level. In practical terms, this means that an educational experience has to guarantee a number of conditions. These are explored in Table 1.2.

Table 1.2 Maslow's hierarchy of needs

Need	Implications for programme design and presentation
Physiological needs (to maintain homeostasis)	
Warmth, food, drink, shelter, sex	Attention to the environment: adequate accommodation, regular refreshment breaks, a reasonable working day
Safety needs (to be free from the threat of aggression, hostility)	
Physical and psychological security	Guaranteeing freedom from external threats (fire, etc.); secure boundaries; no obvious ego threat

Continued

Need	Implications for programme design and presentation
Social needs (to develop a sense of belonging)	
Legitimate membership; community	The opportunity to interact through social exchange (e.g. during registration, but also in opening activities through introductions and an opportunity to share experiences, thinking)
Esteem needs (to develop a sense of self-worth and the capacity to engender that in others)	
Respect, confidence, competence	The opportunity to acquire knowledge and skills and the ability to manifest appropriate attitudes through structured learning interventions with supportive and authentic feedback
Cognitive needs (to know and understand)	
Different levels of cognition • Knowledge • Comprehension • Application • Analysis • Synthesis • Evaluation Different levels of skill acquisition • Perception • Guided response • Mastery • Autonomy Different levels of attitudes • Perceiving • Complying • Accepting • Internalising	Through demonstration, modelling, specific instruction and feedback, learners can move through the levels via: Cognition: types of questions Skills: four-stage approach Attitudes: encourage appropriate affect (e.g. team membership)
Aesthetic needs (to value symmetry, order)	
	A programme that works, for example runs to time, experienced and competent instructors who care about learning – for themselves and others – and fun

Continued

Table 1.2 *Continued.*

Need	Implications for programme design and presentation
Self-actualisation (to be an autonomous individual)	
In touch with reality	An experienced faculty capable of
Acceptance of self and others	manifesting these behaviours as a matter
Spontaneous	of routine gives learners confidence and
Problem solving	also models appropriate behaviour
Tolerance of ambiguity	
Gemeinschaftsgefühl (empathy and compassion)	
Creativity	
Self-transcendence (to develop actualisation among others)	
Concern for others' development	As above
Ego security – not threatened by others' achievements	

Maslow's theory has been criticised for its lack of scientific rigour but it does have some useful things to say about how events can be organised and presented. It is certainly true that unless the basic needs at the bottom of the hierarchy are met, at least to some extent, then learning will be hampered. Accordingly, attention to the conditions within which learning is to take place is essential. More important, however, is the psychological domain within which people will interact with others in a complex, dynamic environment. It is the responsibility of the trainer to ensure that this is a challenging but safe area within which people will learn.

Summary and learning

Adults are usually voluntary learners and need to be actively engaged in their own learning. They need goal-orientated, relevant, practical experiences in order to get the most from teaching. While many admit only to intrinsic motivation the reality is that many external factors affect this as well.

References

Dewey J. *Experience and Education*. Collier Books, New York, 1938.
Knowles M. *The Adult Learner: A Neglected Species*. Gulf Publishing, Houston, 1973.

Kolb DA & Fry R. Toward an applied theory of experiential learning. In: Cooper C, ed. *Theories of Group Process*. John Wiley, London, 1975.

Lewin K. *Field Theory in Social Science: Selected Theoretical Papers*. Harper & Row, New York, 1951.

Malone TW & Lepper MR. Making learning fun: a taxonomy of intrinsic motivations for learning. In: Snow RE & Farr MJ, eds. *Aptitude, Learning and Instruction: III. Cognitive and Affective Process Analyses*. Erlbaum, Hilsdale, NJ, 1987.

Maslow A. *The Farther Reaches of Human Nature*. The Viking Press, New York, 1971 http://chiron.valdosta.edu/whuitt/COL/motivation/motivate.html.

CHAPTER 2

A structured approach to teaching

Learning outcomes

By the end of this chapter you should be able to demonstrate an understanding of:
- The structured approach to teaching
- Set (including environment)
- Dialogue
- Closure

Introduction

This chapter sets out the basic principles of teaching which will be used throughout the guide. These principles can be used to plan and deliver all forms of teaching, whether lectures, discussions, workshops, skill stations or scenarios.

Teaching may be defined as a *planned experience which brings about a change in behaviour*. The important words here are 'planned' and 'change in behaviour.' We all learn from experience, but teaching involves a planned intention to bring about the learning of specified material which will result in a desired outcome.

There are always three stages to consider:

- Set (including environment)
- Dialogue
- Closure

Pocket Guide to Teaching for Medical Instructors, Second Edition. Edited by Ian Bullock, Mike Davis, Andrew Lockey and Kevin Mackway-Jones. © 2008 Blackwell Publishing, ISBN: 978-1-4051-7569-2.

These are discussed in more detail below.

Set (including environment)

The teaching environment is an integral part of the teaching process. All aspects of the environment should be considered. These include heating, lighting, ventilation, acoustics, and the arrangement of the furniture.

The environment can radically affect how a teaching session is conducted and how it will be interpreted by the learners. For example, rows of chairs restrict participation, whereas a circle implies that everyone is expected to contribute. Suboptimal heating and lighting can undermine a teaching session which has otherwise been meticulously prepared. Students who cannot hear the instructor or see the demonstration will have no teaching at all.

The environment must, then, be conducive to the learning that has been planned.

Set is about creating the conditions within which learning can be maximised. It has been described in a number of ways but the essential components need to include:

• Atmosphere
• Motivation
• Objectives
• Roles

These are 'set' in the first few minutes of any session. It is during this time that the instructor will establish the *atmosphere* suggested by the environment and enhance the learners' *motivation* by demonstrating the usefulness of the content for them. During set, the *objectives* will be stated and the learner's and instructor's *roles* will be made clear, for example the learners should be told whether they are to be active or passive, ask questions or participate in other ways.

Practically, then, they need to know who you are; who they are; and what they are going to do during your session. Avoid telling them that '*This is the most important lecture you are going to hear today*' if only to avoid upsetting your colleagues who are to follow. However, it is worth spelling out the significance of the session and how it fits into the programme as a whole. A statement of objectives or learning outcomes provides a useful agenda for the session and gives you something to return to during the final part of the session. Your audience need to have a sense of what their role might be: let them know if you are going to ask them questions or engage in discussions with their neighbours. Tell them if you are willing to take questions during the session or reserve questions for the end. Create an appropriate atmosphere: this is rarely achieved by telling a joke. While it is hoped that your audience will find you engaging and interesting, you are not auditioning for a late night spot in a comedy club. Set prepares the teaching group for learning.

Dialogue

This is the main part of the planned experience, and involves an interaction between learner and teacher that brings about the planned change in behaviour. Dialogue contains the essential subject matter, whether it be a lecture, workshop, discussion or scenario. This represents the central core of the session and will be by far the longest section.

There are many ways of conducting the dialogue – the instructor may lecture throughout, may facilitate a candidate discussion or may use some combination of these. Whatever technique is used the instructor must ensure that the content is available to the learner in a clear and logical form, and at a level which can be understood.

Checking whether the ideas have been understood usually involves questions and answers in one form or another. Giving an appropriate response to the learner's question or comment – a response that promotes learning – is the essence of dialogue.

Closure

The final part of the teaching session should be the closure. A teaching session, which does not end clearly but just peters out not only has an unsatisfactory feel about it, but may also leave unanswered questions in the students' mind. A good closure has three parts:
• Questions
• Summary
• Termination
A period for questions from the students allows any remaining problems to be aired and dealt with. A concise summary pulls together the key points of the session and can relate them to other areas. Finally the termination ends the session. The latter can be

achieved in a variety of ways. The most obvious is direct verbal instruction linked with a break in eye contact and a physical move away from the class.

In the chapters which follow you will find that each mode of teaching is broken down into the three constituent phases – set (including environment), dialogue and closure as discussed above.

Summary and learning

A structured approach can be applied to most teaching interventions. By ensuring that set (including environment) is clear, dialogue is engaging and closure is appropriate the learning experience will be optimised.

CHAPTER 3
Lecturing effectively

Learning outcomes

By the end of this chapter you should be able to demonstrate an understanding of:
- The value of the lecture
- The importance of questions
- What and how you communicate

Introduction

It is extremely likely that sometime during your education you sat in a darkened lecture theatre wondering why you were there. It is unlikely that you learned very much from that experience and you would have to gain access to the lecture content through another medium – usually a book.

At its worst, the lecture is based on a culture of silence – lectures traditionally can be seen and experienced as passive events. It's even been said that a lecture is a process by which the notes of the lecturer become the notes of the student without passing through the mind of either. There is some truth in that. There is, however, a considerable body of evidence that active learning is required if adult learners are going to benefit from an educational intervention. This chapter will explore ways in which a lecture can be interactive, and thereby a more powerful experience for both teacher and learners in order that it is to reach its potential as a learning experience.

Pocket Guide to Teaching for Medical Instructors, Second Edition. Edited by Ian Bullock, Mike Davis, Andrew Lockey and Kevin Mackway-Jones. © 2008 Blackwell Publishing, ISBN: 978-1-4051-7569-2.

The benefits of lectures are usually summarised as follows:
- Disseminating information (possibly to large numbers)
- Reducing the risk of ambiguity
- Stimulating learner interest
- Introducing learners to content/tasks before other instructional processes.

Disseminating information

The lecture has the ability to tell an audience (anything from six to millions – via television transmission) about something. More commonly in continuing medical education, your audience is likely to be relatively small (12–30). Nevertheless, it is an opportunity to give the same message, although without getting some kind of feedback, it is possible that the receivers take something different away with them.

Reducing ambiguity

Lectures rarely break new ground, they are much more likely to provide the opportunity to clarify information that students have learned in other contexts – e.g. reading a text or watching a demonstration. Questions, in both directions, can contribute to this process.

Stimulating learner interest

When you ask people to recall the best lecture they have ever heard, they are more likely to comment on the personal style, charisma and entertainment value of the lecturer rather than its content. What lecturers are doing in these cases is encouraging, albeit subtly, their audience to go away and do some reading and thinking about their subject matter.

Introducing content

Lectures can, therefore, lay the foundations for more detailed study by signposting learners in particular directions.

Lectures have limitations including the inability to teach skills. It is also difficult to present complex and/or particularly abstract ideas. However, the main disadvantage has already been alluded to above: that of attention span. Studies point to different conclusions, ranging from 20 minutes to a maximum of 40 minutes depending on the nature, type and extent of interaction. There is some evidence to suggest that a variety of learner-centred activities can extend this period to 50–60 minutes and some of these will be explored later.

Structure

As shown in Chapter 2, a structure (set, dialogue and closure) can be applied to any teaching session. Lectures are no exception.

Set (including environment)

It is important to check your environment before you are due to give your lecture. Therefore, it is not a good idea to arrive just as your lecture is due to take place. Give yourself time to go to address some important issues.

- *Check the layout*: It is likely that a room will be set up for a lecture (i.e. rows of chairs facing a screen) but someone may have been running a workshop before you, and chairs may be in a circle or horseshoe.
- *Test the projection facilities*: In most cases, you will find a computer and data projector but make sure you are familiar with the computer, where to put your flash drive, whether there is a remote control. For peace of mind, have a backup for your presentation. One way of doing this is to email your presentation to yourself and/or the local organiser.
- *Adjust temperature and lighting*: If the room has been occupied for some time, open windows or run the air conditioning; make sure that your slides are visible with lights on or dimmed.
- *Check for a clock*: If there is not one visible, remind yourself to use your watch. Contrary to opinion, it is not distracting for a lecturer to keep an eye on the time.

Your slides should include learning outcomes or objectives. These serve a number of purposes, including giving your audience a sense of where your session is going. The set is the opportunity you have to claim credibility, by virtue of who you are and what you do. The audience would already have made an assessment of you based on your appearance, but they need to be reassured that you are qualified to be introducing the topic to them. It is not immodest to lay claim to your professional role and your expertise in a particular area. You do, of course, have to live up to the claims you make by being authoritative and knowledgeable.

During the set it is useful to let your audience know what roles they will be expected to fill: whether they can ask questions, whether you will be asking them to engage in any activities. You might like to let them know if you are going to give them handouts or make your presentation available to them electronically. This will determine whether or not they take notes.

Unlike in a wedding speech, you are not required to tell jokes. Unless you have good comic timing, your jokes are appropriate and funny, this can be a high-risk strategy.

Dialogue

Put quite simply, the dialogue is the content and the substance of the learning outcomes you introduced in the set. In some cases, you will be working from pre-prepared slide sets which have an approved content. In other cases, you will be presenting your own slides. Whatever the situation, much of the experience for the audience will be in how you present your information, rather that the what. In fact, some experts argue that only 7% of communication is about the words you speak, as Figure 3.1 suggests.

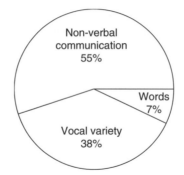

Figure 3.1 Communication skills.

Vocal variety

Vocal variety or verbal style refers to:
- Voice
- Emphasis
- Pace
- Enthusiasm

You might think that there is nothing you can do about your voice, but that is not entirely the case. Pitch and projection are two things which will ensure that your audience can hear you. Certain sections may need emphasis and you will develop a personal style as to how this can be achieved. Strategies range from slowing down, repetition and simply telling the audience that what you are going to say. The pace at which you speak is important even when you are not expecting your audience to take notes. Slightly slower than normal conversation gives your audience time to reflect on what you are saying. Enthusiasm is very contagious as is its opposite. Generally, you should communicate your interest in your subject by speaking about it with a degree of animation. Manic fervour may, however, serve to distract the audience from the content.

Verbal tics can become a distraction to an audience, who focus on how many times you use a word or phrase rather than listening to the content. Common ones are 'OK', 'so ...', 'you know', 'umm'. Linguists call these 'hesitation phenomena', and they are a product of either lack of confidence or working memory capacity. More often than not, speakers are not aware of their tics so it is advisable to get feedback from colleagues.

Non-verbal communication

The 55% of communication that isn't verbal covers a whole range of behaviours including:

- Gesture
- Posture
- Position
- Proximity
- Movement
- Eye contact
- Facial expression

In addition to these, there are other, sometimes subtle, signs that are difficult to make explicit or interpret readily. They often manifest themselves in vague impressions rather than hard data.

Consider the 'Do's and Don'ts' given in Table 3.1.

Words

The words you speak are clearly important and even when you are using course slides, you are in control of what you say. It is never advisable to read or remember a script because you can be sure that you will not engage the audience. If you feel the need for security, you might want to put key words on small index cards. In general, however, the slides should be enough to remind you of what you want to say.

Table 3.1 Do's and Don'ts

	Do	Don't
Gesture	Use natural gestures	Over-exaggerate arm waving
Posture	Look relaxed	Stand rigid; slouch against the wall
Position	Both sides of the room at different times	Hide behind a table or a lectern; stand in the projector beam
Proximity	Close enough	Invade personal space
Movement	Move naturally and purposefully (i.e. to get closer to someone who is asking or answering a question)	Amble aimlessly
Eye contact	Sweep the room at eye level	Gaze at the ceiling or the screen
Facial expression	Look interested; smile	Look bored or irritated
Fixation	Eye contact with the whole room	Get obsessed with someone who answers your first question

Interaction

While these elements are extremely important, some attention has to be paid to the structure of your lecture. As we have already discussed, there are serious limitations on what you can achieve by talking alone. However, there may be opportunities within the lecture format to allow an audience to explore and engage with the ideas in conversation with other learners and you as a teacher. Some of these are outlined in Table 3.2.

Questions

Questions are an important way of achieving dialogue and interactivity. They are, however, not quite as simple as they might appear and a bit of background understanding can help the instructor immensely.

Table 3.2 Interactions within the lecture

	Setting the task	Your response
Opportunities to reflect	Think about what I have just told you. How does it fit in with your previous experience? How might you integrate this new approach in your practice?	Taking contributions from enough people to show that you are interested in what they have to say
Pairs and small group discussion – problem solving, sharing information or experiences	Talk to your neighbour about the last time you met a similar scenario. What might have improved the outcome?	Recording ideas on flip chart
Prioritising, sequencing, sorting	Look at these features on the screen. What order would you deal with these issues in?	Completing a grid on the flipchart – you can be preparing this while they undertake the task

Using questions to determine the level of learning

Bloom *et al.* (1956) describe six levels in the cognitive domain and there are different ways of asking questions in order to elicit the level you want your audience to engage in as follows:

- *Knowledge*: Seeking factual information, for example *In what year was Descartes born?*
- *Comprehension*: Checking understanding, for example *What European intellectual tradition did his work contribute towards?*
- *Application*: Exploring the relevance, for example *How did his work affect that of other scientists and philosophers in the 16th century?*
- *Analysis*: Checking the significance, for example *How could 'cogito, ergo, sum' prove the existence of God?*
- *Synthesis*: Putting knowledge of one subject together with that of another, for example *In what ways was Descartes representative of continental european rationalism as opposed to the empiricism more dominant in British philosophy?*
- *Evaluation*: Comparing with other philosophers, for example *In what ways did Descartes differ from (a) the Socratic tradition? (b) modern philosophers like Wittgenstein?*

Clearly, some of these questions lend themselves more readily to the seminar rather than the lecture theatre – a further reminder of the limitations of the lecture as a teaching modality.

Methods
Regardless of the level of the question, you can ask them in a number of ways:

Open questions, to the group as a whole: This gives everyone the opportunity to demonstrate their knowledge and insight and if the question has been phrased appropriately and at the right level, there is likely to be someone in the audience who will be able to answer it.

Questions to random, named individuals: This is intended to keep an audience on their toes and attentive to what you are saying. It can, however, be intimidating and not just to the new learner. Even experienced members of the audience can sometimes be under considerable pressure and may forget things that they would reasonably be expected to know.

Questions along a row: Asking 10 people to name ten known facts has a number of negative effects: the first person has many options open to them, the second person, one less and so on. By the time you get to the eighth person, there are only three left and pressure along the row will almost certainly guarantee that students will not be able to contribute. In the meantime, students in the first few positions can take a break and possibly lose concentration and a sense of engagement.

Pose, pause, pounce: This is not an uncommon strategy and it has the merit in encouraging all the audience to think of a possible answer before someone (who may look as if they know) is invited to respond.

Whatever the strategy, there are a number of things you need to do in response to an answer, assuming for the moment that it is correct.

Responses
Acknowledge it: Say 'thank you', rather than 'excellent' or any other over-enthusiastic superlative. A reason for this is that answers to (particularly low level) questions are rarely anything other than successfully recalling something from memory – often from another session.

Repeat or paraphrase the answer: some people talk very quietly and other members of the audience may not hear them.

Expand on the response, particularly if it is partial.

Ask supplementary question(s).

Relate it to other parts of your lecture, if relevant.

Consider this exchange:

> *Instructor*: 'Who can tell me what ABC stands for'
> *Student*: 'Airway, breathing and circulation'
> *Instructor*: 'Excellent!'
> *Rest of audience*: ('I knew that!')

compared to:

> *Instructor*: 'What modifications do you have to make to the
> Glasgow Coma Score when dealing with a head-injured
> infant?'
> *Audience*: (thinking about it ...)
> *Student*: 'erm, response to voice ... can't be the same?'
> *Instructor* (nodding and giving eye contact to the respondent):
> 'Yes, response to voice. A small infant or baby could not
> respond articulately to a question. (To the group) Any other
> thoughts?'

Because lectures are rarely introducing new material, and very
rarely, complex or abstract material, the likelihood is that respond-
ents will answer correctly. However, you do need to be prepared
for two phenomena: the wrong answer, and silence.

It is important that you allow both, but the strategies are some-
what different. Consider this:

> *Instructor*: 'Does anyone know the correct dose of amiodarone
> before the 4th shock in a cardiac arrest?'
> *Audience*: (looking at ceiling, fingernails, etc.)
> *Instructor*: 'Anyone?'
> *Student*: '1 mg'
> *Instructor*: 'Well ok, the right answer is 300 mg but you don't
> need to remember that because you can look it up. It is likely
> to be on the wall in the resuscitation room.'
> *Audience*: ('Phew!')

and

> *Instructor*: 'OK. Who can tell me what the energy presence,
> essential for contraction and relaxation of muscle fibres, within
> cardiac muscles is?'
> *Audience*: Silence.
> *Instructor* (after 5 seconds or so): 'Well, that was a difficult one.
> The answer is ATP, Adenosine Triphosphate molecules. The
> way I remember it is that the cardiac muscle fibres are like
> part of an engine, functional units that still need petrol as the
> energy source in order for them to work efficiently. ATP is the
> energy source for cardiac muscles'.

Obviously, there should be variations on these, but you should
look for the supportive, rather than hypercritical or sarcastic.
('Idiot, you think the first shock should be 50 J? I might need to
talk to your clinical director'.) Whatever the strategies you adopt
in the dialogue, you should be aiming for a conversation that enables the audience to share with you and everyone else, a more certain understanding of the issues.

Closure

Closure has three stages: asking for questions (and answering
them); summarising and termination.

Asking for questions (and waiting for 10 seconds to get any),
gives an audience the opportunity to check any uncertainties they
may have. In general, it is safe to treat these as genuine requests
for information and you answer them briefly and succinctly. You
may, however, come across the occasional individual who will ask
something like:

Student: 'I read in a recent edition of the Annals of Emergency
Medicine that ...'

Invariably, this student is trying to impress you and the rest of
the audience, but is unlikely to succeed. However, it is vital that
you do not undermine the student (however you might feel) as
the question may mask uncertainty and a lack of confidence.

The summary is your opportunity to give the students a 'take-
home message' and it should relate directly to the learning outcomes you spelled out in the set. Once more, it should be succinct

and not revisit the whole content of what you have had to say. The summary should always follow questions – this ensures that the lecture does not run over time ('I can accept one more question before I summarise') and also ensures that the audience leaves with your take-home message fresh in their mind rather than an awkward question.

Termination is important because it avoids the situation in which the audience are not sure what is going to happen next. Something like 'Right, wait here as Professor Angstrom is going to talk to you about a new way of thinking about the control of Type 1 diabetes' or 'Thanks for your attention, and now it's time for coffee. Be back by 11.15.' This is much more preferable to the audience sitting uncomfortably while the lecturer shuffles papers or recovers a data stick.

Summary and learning

A lecture is an opportunity to remind people of what they may have come across in other contexts and a chance to share issues and concerns within a safe environment. While lectures are not good at delivering complex knowledge or practical skills, they have a distinct place in learning. Using techniques, such as questioning, to engage learners improves the experience.

References

Bloom B, Englehart M, Furst E, Hill W, & Krathwohl D. *Taxonomy of Educational Objectives: The Classification of Educational Goals. Handbook I: Cognitive Domain*. Longmans, Green, New York, Toronto, 1956.

CHAPTER 4
Teaching skills

Learning outcomes

By the end of this chapter you should be able to demonstrate an understanding of:
- The importance of skills teaching
- The four-stage approach to skills teaching

Introduction

The development and retention of practical skills is of great importance in many areas of professional life. Once a skill has been learnt, regular practice and correct performance are key factors in developing mastery of the skill. Learners arriving on courses often come from varied backgrounds with varied experience, and this is often most apparent by their varied ability to perform the range of key skills.

Acquiring a practical skill is influenced by the retention of factual knowledge, the psychomotor performance and the attitude of the candidate as a learner. The interaction between the candidate and the teaching environment is important in achieving a behavioural change in their practice and mastery of a skill. The whole process is about promoting independent practice of the skill.

The process of changing behaviour is situation dependent (in other words, linked to the candidates' experiences). The key to success here is the instructor's ability to help candidates identify how they can apply new information, skills and attitudes to their everyday clinical practice. This familiarity with the context for learning significantly

Pocket Guide to Teaching for Medical Instructors, Second Edition. Edited by Ian Bullock, Mike Davis, Andrew Lockey and Kevin Mackway-Jones. © 2008 Blackwell Publishing, ISBN: 978-1-4051-7569-2.

enhances the learning of new skills and greatly increases retention (Ausubel, 1968). Once this has been established, the skills themselves are best taught in stages. Acquisition of the skill by the candidate reflects their ability to become increasingly organised as a result of the learning experience.

Researchers have demonstrated that retention of both knowledge and psychomotor skills decline sharply after 4–6 months if they are not practiced. The retention of skills that are regularly used by clinicians is more encouraging. Thus over the last decade, we have seen a significant shift from trying to teach all healthcare professionals all domain skills to a more focused approach on skills that they will use in their normal work. This leads to an increased motivation and desire to learn, with candidates realising the value of new skills, which enable them to function in everyday work situations.

Important principles when teaching practical skills are to:
• Teach progressively from the simple to the complex.
• Teach skills in the order in which they will be used.
• Teach one technique at a time.
• Employ continual reinforcement.
• Follow learning with practice.
• Integrate cognitive and psychomotor learning.
• Encourage confident employment of the skills.

Poor retention of resuscitation skills by learners is attributed in many studies to ineffective teaching. The goal of teaching (or the learning outcome) should be change in the behaviour of the learner; repeated practice will greatly enhance achievement and performance. The four-stage approach is the teaching methodology adopted on provider courses, and is centred on the way information is processed by the candidate, and not just the factual information provided (Bullock, 2001).

Structure

Skills' teaching is based on a universal structure for teaching. As discussed in Chapter 2, this consists of set, dialogue (where a four-stage approach is used) and closure.

Set (including environment)

Preparation of the environment in which the skills are taught is essential if the session is to be successful. Often, several groups are taught in the same room and therefore care must be taken to avoid distractions between groups, either by adequate separation or by the use of screens. Candidates must also have enough room to observe the skill as it is demonstrated. Remember, bodies generate heat and a room containing several groups will soon become hot and stuffy.

As the instructor, it is your responsibility to ensure that you have all the equipment needed to teach the skill. You should ensure that it functions and you know how it works. Arrange the equipment in a realistic manner, removing anything that is not essential.

When the candidates arrive for the session, they must be given clear, realistic learning outcomes. Motivate them by explaining the skill's importance and put it into context within the rest of the course. Finally, identify how the candidates are expected to participate in the session. This is vitally important in skills teaching because the initial approach used may be very different to what they have experienced previously. You are responsible for setting the mood, for motivating the candidates through the learning outcomes for the session and for clarifying the roles, that each will play.

Dialogue

This is the main part of the session where the skill is actually taught using the four-stage approach. Although all methods of education are ultimately about the processing of information, the four-stage approach is orientated specifically towards developing the learner's ability to acquire and operate on information received. This is summarised in Box 4.1.

Box 4.1 Four-stage technique for skills teaching

Stage 1   Demonstration of the skill, performed at real speed
  ↓   with or without speech.

Stage 2   Repeat demonstration with dialogue, providing
  ↓   the rationale for actions.

Stage 3   Repeat demonstration guided by one of the
  ↓   learners.

Stage 4   Repeat demonstration by the learner, and practice
                 of the skill by all learners.

The skills teaching algorithm

Stage 1

> **Animating clinical expertise.** Demonstration of the skill, performed at real speed with or without speech.

In this first stage, the instructor demonstrates the skill as they would normally practice it. In order to create realism, the demonstration is performed in real time, allowing the learner a unique 'fly on the wall' insight into the performance of the skill. No commentary or explanation is given, but any verbalisation that accompanies the skill should be included, for example shouting for help. The demonstration provides the candidate with strong visual imagery which shapes new learning.

Stage 2

> **Reinforcing components of clinical expertise.** Repeat demonstration with dialogue, providing the rationale for actions.

During this stage there is an exchange of facts and ideas between teacher and learner. In stage 2, the instructor is able to slow down the whole performance of the skill, providing the basis for actions and indicating the evidence base for the skill where appropriate. Involving learners by engaging them in dialogue underpins theories of adult learning. Involving the candidate and acknowledging what they bring to the learning environment serves to increase their motivation and desire to learn. This potentially allows the instructor to lead them from what they already know to what they need to know. Provision of meaningful feedback is important to facilitate acquisition of the skill. A period of time for questions within stage 2 can enable the candidates to gain clarity and the instructor to assess understanding prior to stage 3.

Stage 3

> **Part transition of responsibility for the skill from instructor to candidate.** Repeat demonstration guided by one of the learners.

During this third stage the learner talks the instructor through the skill while the instructor performs it. This allows the candidate to 'gather and organise information from the environment in order to form useful patterns, which form the basis of their own future behaviour' (Eggen and Kauchek, 1998). Strong visual reminders will help the candidate recall the skill under the stressful conditions of actual practice.

At this stage the responsibility for the performed skill is moved firmly away from the instructor towards the learner. The emphasis here is on cognitive understanding (knowledge) that will guide the psychomotor activity (performance of the skill) in stage 4. The instructor must ensure that he/she does not lead the candidate, whilst ensuring that the skill is not performed in relative isolation or out of context. It is also important at this and the following stage to correct error or misapprehension. Opportunity for further questions and reflection on the skill adds to the importance of this stage. Positive reinforcement of good practice will enhance the future practice of each individual learner.

Stage 4

> **Independent candidate practice.** Repeat demonstration by the learner, and practice of the skill by all learners.

This stage completes the teaching and learning process. It completes the transference of ability from the expert (instructor) to the novice (candidate), and helps establish the abilities of learners in the particular skill. For virtually all newly learnt skills, a single practice may be insufficient, and all candidates must be encouraged to continue to practice in order to gain further confidence and competence, until mastery is achieved. Once candidates have demonstrated competency in a particular skill, they should be encouraged to maintain this level of performance throughout the rest of the course, reinforcing skilled practice. The strength of using an information processing approach is that it is concerned predominantly with meaningful, purposeful learning as opposed to learning by rote. The learner therefore becomes 'an active investigator of the environment rather than a passive recipient of stimuli and rewards' (Eggen & Kauchek, 1998).

Closure

Hopefully, most of the questions generated during the skills teaching session will have been raised and answered during stages 3 and 4. It is essential that at the end an opportunity be given for final questions to be aired. A summary should affirm achievement of the objectives for the session, linking the skill to the rest of the course and reinforcing its importance and usefulness.

Summary and learning

The theories of skill acquisition described in this chapter provide the instructor with a firm basis for teaching. This well structured and systematic approach allows repeat practice in a safe environment. The opportunity to gain 'protected' practice and experience is an essential ingredient in psychomotor learning (Quinn, 1995).

The four-stage approach to skills teaching on the provider courses represents the dialogue component in this model. The main focus of using this methodology is to effectively transfer skill from the expert (instructor) to the novice (candidate), as the first step towards gaining skill mastery.

References

Ausubel D. *Educational Psychology: A Cognitive View*. Holt, Rinehart and Winston, New York, 1968.

Bullock I. Skill acquisition in resuscitation. *Resuscitation* 2000; **45**: 139–143.

Eggen PD & Kauchek DP. *Strategies for Teachers. Teaching Content and Thinking Skills*. Prentice Hall, Englewood Cliffs, 1998.

Quinn FM. *The Principles and Practice of Nurse Education*, 3rd edn. Chapman and Hall, London, 1995.

CHAPTER 5

Managing role-play and scenarios

Learning outcomes

By the end of this chapter you should be able to demonstrate an understanding of:
- The aims of role-play and scenario teaching
- How to facilitate role-play

Introduction

Role-play and scenario teaching are based on the notion of 'let's pretend ...' or more seriously 'a willing suspension of disbelief' within which learners step outside of their own experiences and try out behaviours, perhaps at the edge of their comfort zone.

There are five common types of role-play:

- *Improvisation*: Learners use their own responses and actions in a given situation; in other words, they behave as themselves but in a novel (to them) context. For example 'You are in the bar at the theatre when an old man nearby clutches his chest and falls to the floor ...'.
- *Structured*: Learners are given a role to play with clear instructions on how this should be performed. For example, 'You are a nervous junior doctor confronted with a febrile child and her mother ...'.
- *Prepared improvisation*: As with improvisation but following a discussion as to the nature of the roles, and possible outcomes.
- *Reverse role-play*: When learners play a role other than their normal one to gain insight into the thoughts, attitudes and behaviours of

Pocket Guide to Teaching for Medical Instructors, Second Edition. Edited by Ian Bullock, Mike Davis, Andrew Lockey and Kevin Mackway-Jones. © 2008 Blackwell Publishing, ISBN: 978-1-4051-7569-2.

others, for example, the learner might play a parent being informed about serious illness in a baby.

• *Exaggerated role-play*: Over-developing the features of a character to make a particular point, for example, an aggressive relative receiving bad news.

Role-play can also be used to teach specific interpersonal skills which may then later be included in more complex simulations. For example, telephone discussions with a senior clinician about a referral may be conducted by seating two learners back-to-back.

As with all teaching modalities, attention has to be paid to planning and facilitation, with attention to environment and set being central to the success of the subsequent dialogue. There are differences between the two, largely arising from the fact that role-plays tend to be free of equipment while scenarios rely on equipment.

Scenarios (sometimes called moulages) are focussed role-play often used in healthcare teaching.

Jones (1987) defines a scenario as:

… an untaught event in which sufficient information is provided to allow the participants to achieve reality of function in a simulated environment.

Presented in these terms, scenario teaching can overcome some of the traditional reservations about this form of teaching by emphasising emotional security (see Maslow in Chapter 1).

Scenarios have the capacity to allow learners to integrate their learning from other contexts: reading, lectures, skills stations and workshops. In something approaching real time, learners can interact within a context, including other health professionals and relevant equipment (ECG, tubes, collars, etc.); with manikins or actors; and with instructors who provide clinical and other information and prompt learners as to the correct way in which to assess a patient and to make decisions in a way that is, as far as possible, true to life.

At the heart of scenario teaching is role-play in which learners act out how they imagine how they may behave in another role in given circumstances.

Structure of a role-play session

Set (including environment)

For most role-play you won't need much more than chairs, possibly supplemented by some equipment to add to the illusion.

Mainly, you need to consider where to place your chairs for the role-players and any observers. Things to consider include:

- *Privacy*: Being overlooked by people external to the immediate group.
- *Proximity*: How close do you want people to be to one another?
- *Eye lines*: Do you want the audience or a critiquer to be in direct eye line with the main role-player?
- *Other furniture*: Would a role-player need a desk or other surface to make notes?

The first three of these relate more to the emotional, rather than the physical environment and because of the nature of the roles that are being explored, this needs thought.

Even though role-play is not *real*, it does need to be *realistic* and this also needs careful planning. Much of that, however, will be built into the design of the role-play and that is beyond the scope of this chapter. Where you can ensure some feasibility, however, is by ensuring that individuals are given roles they could reasonably be expected to play: a junior trainee in Emergency Medicine might struggle to role-play a consultant paediatrician discussing possible child abuse with parents. The role description and the context should be enough to enable the role-players to explore the issues experientially within a constrained period of time followed by shared reflection about what took place.

It is vital that role-play is properly explored in order for everyone (role-players, critiquer and audience) to learn from it. Time management is something that you need to emphasise, so that the role-players know how long they have got and that you will let them know when they need to move towards closure.

Dialogue

During the role-play episode itself, the facilitator is there to listen, and to manage time boundaries. It might be helpful to make notes to assist the discussion that follows, which is also part of the dialogue. While feedback and critiquing is part of this process, the post-episode discussion is where additional learning can take place. During this time, participants should be encouraged to explore thoughts and feelings and to identify problematic and challenging moments. As far as is possible from memory of what is, after all, an ephemeral event, comments and discussion should be based on evidence – what people said, and how they said it. A shared exploration of this can be a powerful learning experience for role-players and observers.

Structure of a scenario session

Set (including environment)

The environment for a scenario is considerably more complex, involving equipment, and decisions about manikins or actors.

Equipment will depend entirely on the nature of the scenario being offered: clearly there will be a difference between what you need for a paediatric resuscitation in an Emergency Department and what you would be looking for in a critical care area. The best way to determine what you need is to 'walk through' the scenario. This will allow you also to make a number of decisions about what is missing and consider questions like what to use if there is nothing to suction with. This process can also alert you to any other uncertainties or ambiguities that are present in the scenario story.

Some issues may arise because of the way in which the manikin functions. While modern, increasingly complex manikins are becoming available much teaching still involves older, less realistic dolls. The detail of the more interactive manikin is beyond the scope of this chapter except to say that instructors must learn how to use them *before* teaching with them.

The use of live patients (actors or real patients) can provide some considerable advantages, but also some disadvantages. These are summarised in Box 5.1.

Box 5.1 Comparison of manikins and real patient or actors

	Manikin	Real patient or actor
Realism		√ √
Appearance	√	√ √
Verbal/physical interaction		√
Procedure performance	√ √	
Safety	√ √	√

Among the difficulties presented by real patients or actors is the need to behave realistically. Thus they need to be carefully briefed and must practice the scenario so that difficulties can be resolved. If they are made up so that they look as if they have the illness or trauma that they are supposed to have, this may add to the learner's experience.

Dialogue

Whether it is a manikin or a real patient, the responsibility for providing accurate patient feedback belongs to the instructor running the scenario. Learners quickly recognise this and look for feedback. It is better, therefore, to be proactive, rather than reactive, thus:

> *Learner* (to helper): 'Could you check blood pressure?'
> (pause)
> *Learner* (to instructor): 'What's the blood pressure?'
> *Instructor*: '90 over 70.'

as opposed to:

> *Learner* (to helper): 'Could you check blood pressure?'
> (pause)
> *Instructor*: '90 over 70.'

In the second example, the instructor is providing clinical information in real time thereby adding to the fidelity of the scenario. The role of the instructor in a scenario is to provide this clinical information and offer the occasional prompt in order to help the learner keep within the protocols. These should be subtle, for example:

> 'What do you think should happen next?'

as opposed to:

> 'Do you think you should move onto circulation now?'

The instructor's other main responsibility is to manage time flow. Some learners may be incredibly slow and they need to be prompted by adding in new, and possibly urgent, clinical signs (e.g. 'the patient is losing consciousness'). Others may move rapidly, usually by telling the instructor what they would do, rather than actually doing it. These can be controlled by simple requests, for example:

> *Learner*: 'I would get in two lines, measure cap refill and get blood pressure'
> *Instructor*: 'Show me'.

Remember, the scenario is an integration of skills and knowledge acquired elsewhere and learners should be encouraged to demonstrate their psychomotor ability as well as their knowledge.

A note on safety

Among the concerns associated with scenario teaching is that of safety, particularly in the context of defibrillation or the safe use/disposal of sharps. Sessions should be terminated immediately in the event of safety being compromised.

Closure

As discussed earlier in this chapter, role-play and scenario teaching have a strong emotional component and participants need to be allowed to return to normal, particularly if they have been dealing with issues which could resonate powerfully with their own experience. This can be achieved very easily by asking them to relate personal details of a trivial nature (e.g. 'So, Alison, where are you going on holiday this summer?'). This serves to remind Alison who she really is.

As with all teaching modalities, role-play and scenarios need to close properly, by:
• Inviting questions or comments about the issues that have emerged.
• Offering a summary of the learning that has taken place – often by revisiting the learning outcomes offered in the set.
• Terminating the session and moving learners on to the next event.

Summary and learning

Role-play and scenario teaching differ from other teaching methods in the way in which, if successful, they relate directly to practice. They utilise skills, knowledge and affect in order to enable learners to explore a simulation of their real world.

As an instructor, you should aspire to make the simulations as real as necessary to maximise the learning experience for all participants.

References

Jones K. *Simulations: A Handbook for Teachers and Trainers*, 2nd edn. Kogan Page, London, 1987.

CHAPTER 6

Facilitating discussions and workshops

Learning outcomes

By the end of this chapter you should be able to demonstrate an understanding of:
- The different ways of facilitating group discussions and workshops
- The relative merits and applications of using closed and open discussion techniques
- The strategies for running workshops effectively
- How to plan group discussions and workshops based on a standardised structure for teaching
- The role of group dynamics
- The management of different learner types

Introduction

Working in groups can be an extremely effective method of learning, particularly for professionals in a multidisciplinary environment. The outcomes of well-organised group activity are almost invariably better than those achieved by even the best individual member working alone. It is also recognised that group activity can be extremely useful in assessing adults' ability to apply theoretical knowledge to practice. To achieve these goals this teaching method requires the teacher to be a facilitator of learning rather than a definitive source of knowledge. The challenge therefore is to create a setting where learners benefit from a more student-centred experience.

Pocket Guide to Teaching for Medical Instructors, Second Edition. Edited by Ian Bullock, Mike Davis, Andrew Lockey and Kevin Mackway-Jones. © 2008 Blackwell Publishing, ISBN: 978-1-4051-7569-2.

As explored in Chapter 1, adults bring a wealth of personal experience to the classroom and it is important to recognise and build on this; group activities allow this far better than many other approaches. As with all educational activities, good planning, organisation and facilitation are required. The ideal group size is less than 12 for discussions and less than 8 for workshops. Participants tend to become inactive and contribute less if the group is larger. This chapter explores the different approaches to group discussions and workshops, providing some ideas for their planning whilst highlighting the skills required in facilitating them. Though the skills used in running workshops and discussions are those of a facilitator, the term 'Instructor' will be used throughout, encompassing the roles of teacher and facilitator.

Effective planning is crucial. The first stage is to clearly define the desired outcomes of the session, as this will determine which type of group session you will run. Table 6.1 offers some guidance on choosing the right format.

Table 6.1 Choosing the right format

Type	Closed	Open
Main aim	Reach a decision	Discuss a range of views
Format	Focused	Divergent
Instructor's key role	Starting and finishing, direction	Starting and finishing, subtly encouraging participation

Examples of topics for each type of session include:
- Closed discussion: 'Defibrillation on safety'
  'Major incident equipment'
- Open discussion: 'Should relatives be present during resuscitation?'

Closed discussions lead to clearly defined answers. They can also include elements of skills and may use equipment. Open discussions do not appear on the timetable of some courses – there are, however, frequent informal opportunities for open discussion during breaks and mentor meetings. In addition, for instructors, the more formal open discussions that are the basis for elements of the faculty meetings occur on a daily basis.

Table 6.2 identifies some of the differences between the instructor's role in closed and open discussions.

Table 6.2 Comparison of instructor role in discussions

Instructor role in *closed* discussions	Instructor role in *open* discussions
• Introduces topic, usually stood next to flip chart or OHP	• Introduces topic, usually from a seated position within the group
• Establishes and maintains the 'chair' role	• Relinquishes the 'chair' role
• Outlines the task and learning outcomes	• Facilitates open (not 'through the chair') discussion
• Canvasses opinions systematically	• Allows discussion to flow and develop where possible
• Records opinions	• Encourages elaboration and development
• Carries discussion from one participant to the next	• Encourages reflection on personal experience
• Maintains the group's focus • Allows all to contribute whilst acknowledging, and, where necessary, controlling any candidate behaviours likely to disrupt the group	• Allows all to contribute whilst acknowledging, and, where necessary, controlling any candidate behaviours likely to disrupt the group
• Uses body language and voice for control	• Mainly uses body language for control

Structure of a closed discussion session

Set (including environment)
Apart from the usual considerations of heat, light, comfort, the environment element of set is primarily concerned with seating layout and where the relevant audio visual aid is positioned. Common aides used to focus the discussion are the flip chart, whiteboard or overhead projector. The usual rules apply when using these, but the instructor should be clear about what content will be written, or what pre-prepared content will be revealed and when.

Figure 6.1 shows a suggested layout for seating in a closed discussion that enables all candidates to see and contribute whilst allowing the instructor to maintain control. The instructor sets the mood by saying what is expected of candidate participation before stating clear learning outcomes and commencing the dialogue.

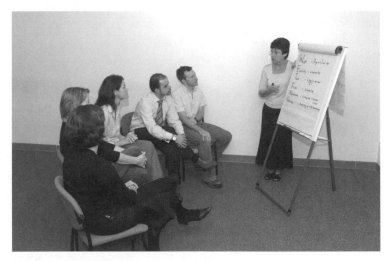

Figure 6.1 Closed format.

Dialogue

The most common pitfall for the instructor in closed discussions is the temptation to deliver a lecture to a small group. The key, therefore, is to ensure candidate participation by engaging them in a non-threatening way and allowing all candidates equal opportunity to contribute, acknowledging that contribution and how it meets the outcomes for the session. The simplest way to engage candidates is to use questions to elicit a response. There are several strategies to consider when asking questions to a group, but a few simple techniques will help get the right result.

Start off by asking a question to the group as a whole before asking one of the candidates (who appears to know the answer) for their response. If it is the right response, acknowledge that fact and write it up if appropriate. When given an incorrect answer re-pose it or refine it and offer it again either to the whole group or the same individual depending on circumstances. This approach to questioning is commonly referred to as the 'pose, pause, pounce' technique. You pose the question, wait for a response then choose an individual to answer, remembering to reflect the answer back to the group. Eye contact is useful if you want to elicit a response from an individual, as it is a powerful way of non-verbally involving the entire group. If a group or individual is reticent, using candidates' names can also be a powerful tool to ensure contribution, for example 'Name one of the 4 H's ... Annie'.

> A good dialogue phase involves all of the candidates, allowing them to reach the learning outcomes for the session within the given time.

Closure
The usual procedure applies. Ask if there are any questions before summarising. It is particularly useful if you refer back to the candidate contributions during your summary, thereby acknowledging their input and reinforcing the learning outcomes. A clear termination is essential here as discussion may continue.

Structure of an open discussion session

Set (including environment)
Again, seating is the main initial consideration. Figure 6.2 suggests a format where a circle of chairs implies equality within the group and the instructor sits within the group. Communication is easier in this arrangement and it also serves to convey a sense of equality. The inclusion of a gap within the seating allows individuals to leave the group with minimal disruption, should that prove necessary. Once the group is assembled, the instructor clarifies the purpose of the discussion and identifies the learning outcomes. These will be exploratory in nature and will describe the group's process

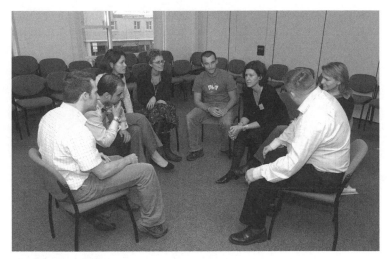

Figure 6.2 Open format.

rather than its conclusions. Occasionally, in open discussions there may be a need to establish ground rules, which can include:
• Confidentiality
• The need to treat the opinions expressed with respect
• One contribution only to be made at any one time.

Dialogue

In contrast to a closed discussion, the instructor does not lead the dialogue, it is driven from within the group. The instructor will need to facilitate the group to keep it on track but should keep contributions to a minimum. The instructor must ensure that everyone is invited to contribute without forcing them to do so. Controlling techniques for verbose or reticent candidates become vital to maintaining control and these are explored later in this chapter. Good non-verbal communication skills may be required to facilitate an open discussion effectively.

Closure

In this instance it may not be appropriate to ask if anyone has any questions, but the instructor should ensure that the session is satisfactorily terminated. If the discussion was particularly heated or if there appear to be some unresolved issues, these should be dealt with before terminating the session. Summary may not be required as there may have been no clear outcomes. However, the instructor should close the session by thanking the group for their contributions.

Workshops

The workshop is an extension of the closed discussion format. Set, dialogue and closure as discussed above remain central to the organisation of workshops. The aim of any workshop is to engage a group of people in study. Many workshops encourage the learner to take part both mentally and physically. Workshops can be organised as a group discussion around a manikin or other audio visual aids (see Figure 6.3) and usually work well if the candidates are in groups of less than eight.

One of the keys to success is to allow the candidates to think through the information supplied for the workshop and confer with their colleagues before reaching a consensus of opinion on

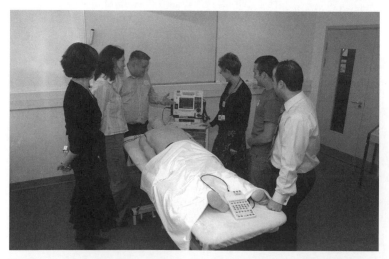

Figure 6.3 Workshop.

how to proceed. At best, the workshop can be a really dynamic process with elements of discovery learning fostering a real sense of achievement for the candidates. At worst, the workshop can turn into a lecture around a set of charts. The good instructor will set clear learning outcomes, give clear guidance on required outcomes and allow the group time and space to reach their conclusions, interjecting where necessary to keep the candidates focused. For example, when using case-based scenarios additional information can be introduced when a particular stage has been reached or to help out when a problem is encountered.

Ideally, a workshop is an opportunity to develop practical skills in a simulated situation and link theory with practice. During the workshop there is the temptation to interject or stand over a group that is working through the task. Sometimes this is necessary if the group lacks direction or is unclear about the task. Some groups, if they require it, will allow a space for the instructor to facilitate causing minimal disruption. Generally it is better if, once the task is set, the groups are allowed to get on with it. Praise can be given during the feedback if a group has worked particularly well together. The important thing to remember is that the workshop is designed to increase the confidence of candidates in applying theoretical principles and developing clinical competence. It also offers the instructor an opportunity to evaluate the impact of the structured learning experience across the range of abilities within the group. One way of facilitating a workshop is to take an approach which has problem-based learning (PBL) as the central theme. This works particularly well in case-study based workshops where the skilled instructor can use the existing knowledge within group to reach sometimes quite complex clinical decisions. This acknowledgement of existing knowledge is a central tenet of adult learning and if used effectively serves to give some ownership of the workshop to the candidates making them work more cohesively and efficiently as a group. The key to this approach is to set a scenario, give relevant clinical information and ask 'What actions should you, as the medical team, take, based on the information so far?' Set the task to the group and give clear time scales for them to report back to the instructor who will interject as necessary to ensure that the correct treatment strategies are clearly identified.

Group dynamics and candidate behaviour

Managing discussions and workshops can be quite complex (Davis, 2006). The instructor's role is to pose the problem and allow students to explore their understanding. They should have read the manual and the purpose is to check their understanding through discussion amongst themselves. The role of the instructor is more of a facilitator during these sessions. This means that you will probably listen much more than you will talk. After your initial statement, you should, through subtle use of body language and a particular approach to asking questions (see below), allow the conversation to develop among the candidates, having them speaking to one another, rather than directing everything to you. This saves you from occupying a judicial role, which is something that can be observed in adult education settings where sessions become:

... emotional battlegrounds with members vying for recognition and affirmation from each other and from the discussion leader.

(Brookfield, 1993)

This is the socio-emotional component of the learning environment and unless it is well handled, can interfere with effective learning for many group members. More significantly, however, it is the nature of the interactions that is expected among the group. The question we should consider is: What is the nature of the intellectual activity that candidates are engaging in? In lectures, this is relatively straightforward: candidates listen, consider, compare with existing knowledge and either accept or reject the conclusions – usually the former. In discussion, however, it is not simply a matter of rehearsing what has been previously read. As Candy puts it:

If cognitive process are indeed processes of reconstruction rather than replicating or depicting an a priori existing reality, then the focus of any explanatory effort must shift from what there is or may be to how we arrive at the conceptual constructs we actually have.

(Candy, 1991)

The strategy to develop this is, as stated above, asking appropriate questions. Mackway-Jones and Walker (1999) help us out here.

As was explored in Chapter 3, appropriate questions are there to reflect the levels of knowledge that candidates might reasonably expect to have:
- Knowing – identify, name, describe
- Understanding – compare, distinguish, show
- Applying/analysing – specify, demonstrate, hypothesise
- Synthesising – create, speculate, design
- Evaluating – assess contribution of differing perspectives.

Discussions and workshops should focus more on understanding and the other higher levels.

Body language

As explored in Chapter 3, some experts in communication argue that body language communicates more than words. Certainly some unconscious behaviours can communicate very effectively and particular attention needs to be paid to these to avoid negative impact on the group. Some helpful strategies include:
- Make frequent sweeps of the group at eye level but do not give eye contact to a person who is speaking. This might sound hostile or aggressive but it makes people speak to the group rather than to you.
- Sit back after your initial statement and subsequent questions.
- Don't validate (nodding, 'excellent') contributions – doing this will encourage the group to believe they have found the right answer and the discussion will have come to an end without all candidates having had time to contribute and to think it through. Again this may feel uncomfortable but it does encourage the group to continue to explore the issues.

Potential issues

The issue that is of most concern to facilitators of interactive sessions is that of control: that if the group is encouraged to talk amongst themselves, instructors will lose control and chaos will reign. This is usually down to expectations/fears about certain candidate types and these have been summarised as talkers, non-talkers and destroyers (Mackway-Jones & Walker, 1999). Destroyers are extremely rare, the other two more common.

You want people to talk; if some people talk too much you can control them readily by:

- Not giving eye contact (see above)
- Turning away slightly so you are orientated towards another part of the group
- Raising an open palm (see Figure 6.4)

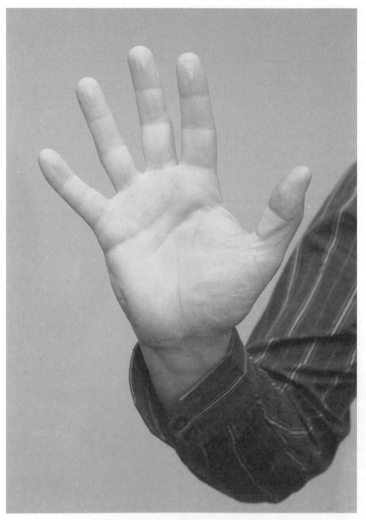

Figure 6.4 Raising an open palm.

- Asking 'What do other people think?'
- Saying 'Hang on a second, [name]'.

It takes a determined talker to continue over the top of those cues. Non-talkers can be encouraged by:

- Giving eye contact
- Turning towards that person
- Offering an open palm (see Figure 6.5)

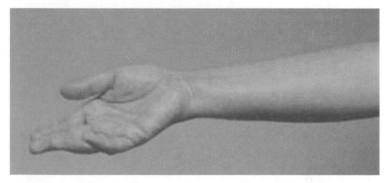

Figure 6.5   Offering an open palm.

- Asking 'Does anyone on this side of the room have any experience'
- Saying '[name], as an ED registrar, you must have come across similar cases'.

Small groups lay bare some of the complex socio-psychological issues of teaching and learning, mainly arising from instructors' concerns about power and authority. However, much of the research suggests that among fairly well motivated communities, group cohesion and a sense of responsibility almost guarantee the status quo: that is, the instructor is the site of power in the group and all group members subscribe to that because of their psychological need for safety.

Summary and learning

Closed discussions, open discussions and workshops are all essentially learner-orientated activities. Each requires slightly different behaviours from the instructor and their learner. The instructor should therefore be attuned to the dynamics within the learning group, exercising control or discretion as necessary. Problems with group dynamics are best dealt with at mentor/mentee meetings where this specific subject can be raised for discussion if deemed necessary. Similarly, problems with individuals who become disruptive or non-engaging within the group may best be dealt with by the group itself if they are empowered to do so. Individual feedback, may also afford opportunities for candidates to reflect on their contribution to group work and dynamics.

References

Brookfield S. Through the lens of learning: how the visceral experience of learning reframes teaching. In: Boud D, Cohen R & Walker D, eds. *Using Experience for Learning*. SHRE/Open University, Buckingham, 1993: 24.

Candy P. *Self-direction for Lifelong Learning*. Jossey-Bass, San Francisco, 1991: 273.

Davis, M. Facilitating interactive discussions. In: Garrioch, M. ed *IMPACT: ill medical patients' acute care and treatment* (second edition). Federation of Royal Colleges of Scotland/Royal College of Anaesthestists.

Mackway-Jones & Walker. *Pocket Guide to Teaching for Medical Instructors*. BMJ Books, London, 1999.

CHAPTER 7

Getting assessment right

Learning outcomes

By the end of this chapter you should be able to demonstrate an understanding of:
- What is meant by assessment and its purpose
- Different assessment approaches
- How assessment may facilitate learning and predict candidate performance

Introduction

Assessment is one of the most challenging aspects of the education process. It typically provokes high emotional responses from both teachers and learners. It is essential that instructors have a basic understanding of assessment methodology and a good understanding of the particular assessment approaches used on courses, so that assessment tools are properly used. This will help increase the reliability of assessments actually reflecting the learner's ability (Perkins, 2001). The purpose of this chapter is to define the educational principles that lie behind the assessment techniques used.

What do we mean by assessment?

In education, the term assessment is used to describe the process of evaluating or making a judgement about a student's ability. This process involves collecting data, observing and measuring

Pocket Guide to Teaching for Medical Instructors, Second Edition. Edited by Ian Bullock, Mike Davis, Andrew Lockey and Kevin Mackway-Jones. © 2008 Blackwell Publishing, ISBN: 978-1-4051-7569-2.

performance and interpreting information about the outcome of an educational process. This can be focused on an individual or on a group of candidates.

The methods of assessment used are based on principles well defined in educational practice, and involve the evaluation of the candidate's performance against pre-set criteria. Both written and practical assessments of knowledge and skills can be undertaken; in all cases the assessor is required to make a judgement about the candidate's performance. The outcome will be more consistent and reproducible when the answer is clear-cut as in a multiple choice question (MCQ) paper. In practical skills the assessment depends more on a subjective opinion that the assessor makes about the candidate's abilities. Assessors need to understand very clearly their own responsibilities in the process as well as the issues that the candidates themselves face. The qualities of an expert assessor have been described by Laryea, 1994:

You need a sense of fairness and willingness to treat people as candidates and not entities. You should not behave in a manner that may create anxiety in the individual that you are assessing. You are not there to fail a person, but to help them realise their potential.

Given this description, the challenge is to ensure that the assessment process actually measures effectively what it is supposed to. In other words, within the context of a training course, it is fit for the purpose of predicting how the candidate will react in a real situation. To achieve this, assessment methods need to be:

- Practically based – real
- Replicable – quality assured
- Affirming – builds confidence
- Enabling – reinforces ability in order to reproduce performance.

The reason for a balanced assessment strategy is to accommodate not just learning behaviours and preferences, but also to match the test experience to what is being observed. Thus, combinations of assessment approaches are used to achieve valid, reliable and feasible tests of attitude, skills mastery, decision making and competence.

Why assess?

The reasons why we assess are:

- to quantify or measure candidate achievement
- to focus and motivate the candidate
- to measure the effectiveness of teaching and learning
- feedback for the student and teacher
- to predict candidate performance when in work-based situations.

The purpose of assessment is to gain insight into (measure) candidate ability in order to ensure that a standard has been reached. The successful attainment of the overall standard does not grant a qualification or license to practice, but does show that competency has been achieved. An important feature of assessment is that candidates receive feedback about their abilities, progress and competence to allow reflection and further professional development planning.

What to assess?

Most courses held for healthcare practitioners involve the acquisition of both knowledge and psychomotor skills. The development of the interpersonal skills necessary to lead or contribute effectively to the overall care plan is also important. Problems may arise during assessment because:

- the scientific basis on which practice is based changes
- the accepted standard may appear unclear or open to individual interpretation
- the candidate is unaware that they are being assessed
- the candidate is unaware of what is being assessed.

It is an important principle that both candidates and those undertaking their assessment are clear about precisely what is being evaluated and what constitutes satisfactory performance. This should cover all the important areas and candidates must demonstrate certain key attributes or minimum standards if they are to complete the course successfully. Those who demonstrate outstanding abilities may be recognised as potential instructors and invited to attend an instructor course.

Examples of assessments used on many courses include:
- Knowledge (MCQ paper)
- Skills performance (continuous assessment)
- Managing complex cases (scenarios).

How to assess

Getting assessment right is a key aim for instructors, and perform-ance here is as important as delivering a good lecture, facilitating a workshop or creating a simulated clinical environment. Candidates should feel confident that decisions reached during assessments are consistent and fair. The following have been identified as particu-larly important in achieving this goal:

Validity, which is concerned with the content of the examination:
- Are the right things being assessed?
- Is the assessment a fair test?
- Does success in the assessment predict good future performance?

Reliability, which is concerned with the accuracy of the assessment:
- Is the assessment passing and failing the right candidates?
- Do different instructors agree with each other?
- Would the candidate obtain a similar result if re-tested without additional learning?

Specificity, which relates to the method of assessment chosen:
- The assessment should be relevant to the skill or area of learning being assessed.
- Simulation is appropriate for developing skills and attitudes whilst evaluating their acquisition.

Feasibility, which is the balance between reliability and validity measured against practical assessment issues (time and resources available)

Fidelity, which is the closeness to reality of the assessment experience:
- The assessment must be as realistic as possible.

When to assess

Both summative and formative approaches are criterion referenced and measure candidate competency against predetermined standards.

There is increasing emphasis on realistic assessment and a move away from short tests of competence that are not necessarily

> **Summative assessment (e.g. MCQ)**
> Assessment using a single testing approach of learning that has taken place and counts towards an overall mark at the end of the period of study.
>
> **Continuous assessment (e.g. skills)**
> An ongoing process throughout the duration of the course, involving repeated sampling of a candidate's practice, providing more realistic assessment. Skills are initially assessed using outcome-based methods and then repeatedly observed throughout the course.

predictive of long-term performance. This is an important shift towards finding and using the best way of predicting and monitoring performance in practice, albeit in a simulated setting.

The opportunity and strength that continuous assessment provides is for multiple interventions targeted at specific behaviour that serve to promote a result in positive behaviour change (Jarvis, 1995). This enables the faculty to further develop the candidates towards the desired level of competency during the course rather than failing them outright for a single poor performance.

How to interpret?

The results of assessment may be expressed by comparing the performance of a candidate with others (i.e. norm referenced) or with defined criteria (i.e. criterion referenced). The latter is considered more appropriate for life support courses.

How to respond?

Assessment should be embedded within the learning process for the candidate, and for this to occur, feedback is essential. For a detailed exploration of this see Chapter 8. The candidate needs to know how they have performed and how they can improve.

Feedback should be specific, constructive, measured and honest. It should be provided as close in time to the assessment as possible. In one off assessments of competence, the candidate needs to know whether they have been successful or not. When dealing with success, praise is clearly appropriate. If they have been unsuccessful then the offer of remedial support is essential and feedback on what they did wrong needs to be supported by feedback indicating how they can correct it.

Failure to pass a course does not necessarily mean that the candidate has failed to learn. Many candidates with the right support and approach will benefit and learn a great deal, and their practice may improve in consequence. Assessment is not and should not be made a measure of a candidate's worth in their occupational role; it is merely a reflection of their ability to demonstrate specific learning outcomes in a particular way at a particular time. Being able to do this is as much about the ability of the instructor to teach as it is of the candidate to learn.

Summary and learning

The assessment of candidates is a fundamental part of an instructor's role. Its purpose is to facilitate the process of learning and to ensure that high standards are maintained.

Assessment should be carefully planned to reflect the content and teaching approach within the curriculum. Getting assessment right facilitates both the candidates' personal and professional development. Enabling instructors to understand and develop confidence in assessment is an important element in measuring the quality of the candidate experience and the course undertaken.

References

Jarvis P. *Adult and Continuing Education: Theory and Practice*. Routledge, London, 1995.

Laryea P. In: Parsloe E, ed. *Coaching, Mentoring and Assessing: A Practical Guide to Developing Competence*. Kogan Page, London, 1994.

Perkins GD, Hulme J & Tweed MJ. Variability in the assessment of advanced life support skills. *Resuscitation* 2001; **50**(3): 281–286.

CHAPTER 8
Giving feedback

Learning outcomes

By the end of this chapter you should be able to demonstrate an understanding of:
- The nature and role of critiquing
- How to give effective feedback

Introduction

Critiquing has increasingly become part of good educational practice because of the opportunity it provides for learners to receive quality feedback on an aspect of their performance. Effective critiquing depends on feedback and disclosure. It is worth taking a moment to look at the theory that underpins these. Figure 8.1 illustrates the concept of the 'Johari Window' (named after its creators – Joseph Luft and Harry Ingham). This illustrates that we know some things about ourselves and are blind to others. Equally, some of our behaviour is apparent to other people and some is not. Thus, four domains exist – an open area: known to ourselves and others, two partially known areas either not known to others (hidden from them) or not known to ourselves (we are blind to it but others are aware of it) or a completely unknown area which is unknown to either ourselves or others.

At the beginning of a feedback session very little information is revealed and, only the open area is available to everybody. In the hidden area (quadrant three) are attitudes, perceptions and facts which only the learner who is being critiqued knows. There are,

---

Pocket Guide to Teaching for Medical Instructors, Second Edition. Edited by Ian Bullock, Mike Davis, Andrew Lockey and Kevin Mackway-Jones. © 2008 Blackwell Publishing, ISBN: 978-1-4051-7569-2.

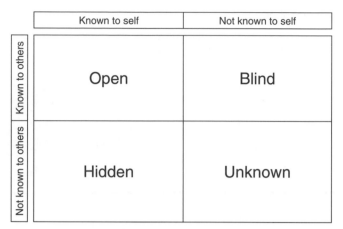

Figure 8.1 The Johari Window (Luft, 1970).

however, aspects of personality, attitudes and events described which the candidate is blind to even though these are apparent to the instructor. Consider for a moment someone you know who is blind to an aspect of their personality or behaviour. It could be someone who talks too much without realising that it is a problem for other people, or someone who constantly says 'Ok'. Whilst thinking of someone else is a relatively easy task, it is much harder to apply the same lens to ourselves – this is where we need other people. Thus, feedback can be extremely useful in pointing out what we do not know about ourselves and highlighting what might benefit from changing. It is the task of an effective critiquer and a willing candidate to reduce the size of the blind and hidden areas – bringing out into the open area (quadrant one) relevant and useful information. On rare occasions the unknown area (quadrant four) reduces – the moment of insight may be uncomfortable for both parties but it can be extremely rewarding for all members of the group.

Feedback methods

In order for feedback and disclosure to occur and be effective the critique process needs to be sensitive, relevant and useful. A number of formulae have been advocated for critiquing. Some of these are outlined in Boxes 8.1–8.3.

Box 8.1 The positive sandwich critiquing model

The positive sandwich
• Tell them what they did well.
• Tell them what they could improve.
• Re-iterate what they did well, ending on a positive note.

Box 8.2 The reflective critiquing model

The reflective model
• Ask them what they feel went well, or were pleased about.
• Respond and tell them what you think went well.
• Ask them what they would like to improve.
• Tell them what you think they could do differently.

Box 8.3 The narrative approach to critiquing

The narrative approach
• Start with the beginning of the experience and talk it logically through with the learner.
• Constantly seek learner's memory of the event, feelings and responses.
• Focus on strengths as well as highlighting ways to improve.

The one that you will have seen most commonly used is the reflective model, sometimes referred to as 'Pendleton's Rules' (Pendleton *et al.*, 1984). It aims to encourage learners to self-assess their strengths and weaknesses whilst expecting the instructor to maintain a fairly rigid formula.

Each of these approaches has its strengths and weaknesses but none of them work well if a number of factors are not included in the instructor's *approach* to giving feedback. Essential elements include:
• Credibility
• Authenticity
• Empathy
• Mutual dialogue.

Credibility

As an instructor who will give candidates a critique on their performance, it is essential that you have credibility. By explaining who you are and why you are the right person to run the teaching session you should establish your credibility at the beginning of a session. Credibility will not automatically be maintained if you do not retain the respect of the learners and demonstrate thoughtfulness about the subject in hand.

Credibility can be interpreted as simply demonstrating knowledge about the subject which is being critiqued. You may have observed instructors making frequent use of examples from their own experience: comments such as, 'When I get into that situation I find it useful to ...' This is an important aspect of credibility: showing that you have the experience and that you have experimented with different styles. It is crucial, however, not to overwhelm learners with your own personal experience when they are deep within the aftermath of the recent scenario. As a critiquer you need to spend more of your time listening rather than talking and this is often much more of a challenge than it sounds.

Above all, credibility is about being precise and being truthful. There is little point in giving feedback which lacks honesty. Critiquing is at its best when it is neither brutal nor too 'touchy-feely'. Candidates often want clear guidance on what their mistakes are and respect honesty above a formulaic approach. It is beneficial to avoid such blanket statements as, *'That was excellent'* because it is rarely helpful or accurate. It is far more useful to make specific points based on what was observed and give suggestions that are concrete and achievable.

There is a significant difference between the following approaches to the same issue as shown in Boxes 8.4 and 8.5.

Boxes 8.4 and 8.5 Two different approaches to critiquing

'The way you laid out all of the equipment was messy and you couldn't find what you wanted.'	'It might work better if you lay the equipment out in a logical ABC approach so that you can find everything when you need it. Is that something that would work for you?'
Box 8.4	**Box 8.5**

There are a number of advantages to the second approach:
- The critiquer offers a practical suggestion of how to improve rather than a comment on what is defective.
- By inquiring into the other person's point of view the critiquer shows that they are listening and prepared to respond.
- The critiquer gains the other person's opinion on what is or is not possible for him as an individual. A dialogue can then take place in which a solution to the problem emerges from either of the two protagonists or from another member of the group. In this situation, it is important not to hold onto your own suggestion and value it above the others. The individual being critiqued needs to have the space to choose the most appropriate and manageable new behaviour.
- The second approach uses a technique known as advocacy with inquiry. Advocacy is when you state what you think rather than expecting the candidate to guess your point of view. Inquiry then gives them the opportunity to respond. Further examples of advocacy with inquiry are given in Box 8.6.

Box 8.6 The use of advocacy with inquiry

- 'At that point I thought X was going on, *what did you think was happening?'*
- 'When the patient collapsed it took you 2 minutes to initiate CPR. *What was going through your mind at the time?'*
- 'I am wondering if … *does this sound like a possibility?'*
- 'When you said X, I thought you meant Y. *How did you intend me to interpret it?'*

It is sometimes stated that critiquing needs to be both tactful and diplomatic. The danger with tact and diplomacy is that they sometimes mean using leading questions because of:
- a desire not to hurt the other person;
- an inability to deal with that hurt;
- not wanting to give a difficult truth.

Consequently, we devise ways to get them to discover it themselves. Hence, we ask leading questions such that (if they work out what our subtext is) they can work out what the problem is *without us ever having to admit it*. We can then pat ourselves on the back for getting the result that we wanted (and controlling the dialogue) and we can describe the learner as having insight. The learner meanwhile may feel manipulated and defensive. We thus inadvertently define insight as the learner agreeing with what the critiquer is saying; but it may be helpful to your learners if you have a broader definition and accept what comes from others. The more accepting and real we are as facilitators, the more open and insightful learners are able to be.

Authenticity

The need for integrity and authenticity is apparent throughout the entire critiquing process and is shown through careful listening, through genuine responses whether puzzlement, distaste or laughter and through precise rather than sloppy use of language. There are certain phrases, which create an impression that the critiquer is not authentic. They can be referred to as platitudes as they are over-used and lack mindfulness. It is important to be attentive to language and to the effects that different words have.

One example of a platitude occurs after a critique by someone else, '*I concur with everything that's been said so far*'. This, like, '*That was excellent!*' is a blanket statement which smothers a mass of information and may serve to belittle both the specifics of what has been done and also comments that have been made. In order to avoid platitudes we must each find our own language and vary what we say by tailoring it to the individual. Being given feedback is potentially very uncomfortable and intensely personal. The instructor needs to remember this, treat each candidate as an individual and maintain an atmosphere in which learning can occur.

'*We all do it*' is another phrase to avoid, partly because we don't all do it and partly because it is tired. Be authentic in acknowledging your faults and be direct focussing on the learner's strengths and weaknesses.

Sometimes a critique sounds like that demonstrated in Box 8.7.

Box 8.7 Relentless optimism

'Tell me what went well with that scenario'.
'Nothing, it was awful!'
'No it wasn't, there were lots of good things about it. Tell me what was good'.
[silence]
'Well I can think of lots of good things'.

This relentless optimism, sometimes in the face of overwhelming evidence to the contrary, occurs because of the belief that a critique must be positive. In addition, a rigid adherence to a formula, at the expense of authenticity, dialogue and learning compounds a delicate situation. Pendleton's rules *are* useful in encouraging novice critiquers to note what is good as well as what might need improving. And being positive is helpful. However, the learners are adults and highly trained in the art of spotting insincerity. Interestingly, repeated requests to focus on the positive, rather than encouraging the candidate, have the adverse effect to that intended: an increasingly demoralised learner with slumped shoulders who avoids eye contact.

The question we need to ask is: how do we find that which is genuinely positive when something has not gone well? There are two issues here: the first is about maintaining our integrity – candidates find it hard to continue to trust an instructor who has been less than truthful because of a desire to remain positive. And the second is that we must ensure that learning occurs, that errors are corrected and that the learner is in a frame of mind to be able to listen, evaluate, interact and suggest alternative strategies.

There are a number of ways in which it is possible to be positive whilst combining the four elements of credibility, authenticity, empathy and mutual dialogue.

1 Be positive about the learning that can occur.
2 Acknowledge how the candidate must be feeling and their desire to improve.
3 Praise helpful suggestions for improvement and the candidate's own perception of errors.
4 Listen attentively to the candidate, support them and show that you value their personal reflections.

Empathy

Empathy, distinct from pity or sympathy, is about acknowledging that the situation the candidate is in might be difficult, stressful and embarrassing. If the instructor can have some level of emotional resonance with the candidate, this understanding will enhance the critique process. In order to do this you sometimes need to look at the situation from their frame of reference rather than your own. Empathy will increase your skill at instinctively working out what is going on behind the actions and words. Recalling your own experiences of being a learner or being given feedback may increase your empathy. Another strategy is to observe the learner's non-verbal cues closely and pick up what they might be feeling. It is however worth checking out with the other person in case you have misinterpreted the cues (Box 8.8).

Box 8.8 Using empathy within a critique

'That looked really difficult. Can you tell me what you felt your main challenge to be there and we'll see if we can work out some alternative strategies you could have tried? Does that sound useful?'

'It looks to me like you are feeling pleased with the way that went. Is that an accurate assessment?'

Empathy has to be genuine and is apparent when we are neither judgemental nor patronising. The moment you as the facilitator stop trying to force the learner into your frame and empathise with the learner's frame, acknowledging their constraints as real, it becomes possible for learning and change to occur. Performing in front of colleagues and being critiqued is a phenomenally stressful situation for the learner, which can be made worse by insensitive critiquing.

It is important then to create a safe environment from the moment the educational encounter begins. Safety is enhanced by the physiological needs being met: heating, lighting, refreshments, breaks; and by attending to the learners' need to feel secure. Maslow (1987) defines some of the safety needs as, *'a freedom from fear, anxiety and chaos [and] a need for structure'*. In addition, security appears to be enhanced by having your contributions valued and accepted, by well-placed humour and by consistency.

You may have observed at times that a critique degenerates into a list (Box 8.9).

Box 8.9 When a critique becomes a list

'You did your calculations, then you evaluated the patient with an ABC approach. You put the oxygen on and got the nurse to call for help...

You started the clock and then checked the baby's heart rate, tone, colour and breathing. When the baby wasn't breathing you used a T-piece...'

That is not a critique, it is a list. Inherent within the word 'critique' is an element of passing some form of judgement. A list is nothing more than a list – you did this, then this, then this. The candidate may not learn anything from this approach.

If you choose to take the narrative approach to critiquing then the information needs to come from the candidate about what they did but the importance really lies in working out why they did it and finding out about their thinking. This may give the instructor the opportunity to work out when and why something went wrong without making assumptions, which are quite likely to be wrong. The type of questions that might help with this approach are:

- 'So tell me, what was the first thing that happened? Then what happened next?'
- 'What was going through your mind at the time?'
- 'Can you recall how that decision was made?'
- 'What prevented you from doing X?'

Mutual dialogue

Being led by a formula such as Pendleton's rules can create artificiality of process and discourage dialogue. If the facilitator strictly polices responses and organises who is to speak when and whether they are to be positive or not then spontaneity is squashed and comments cannot always be made at the appropriate time. Be aware when running a critique and involving others that it is important that it becomes a conversation in which people listen and respond to each other.

In order to engage in mutual dialogue there are several techniques which we need to avoid. The first is talking too much ourselves. We do have knowledge to give, but our best asset is drawing the right learning for the candidate out of them and we cannot know what this will be. Note the difference between this strategy and leading questions where we pre-determine the learning. This is constructivist learning, a process whereby each individual constructs his or her own learning dependent upon prior experiences, learning style and their current frame of mind. Where learners self-identify errors and alternatives in a supportive environment they will probably retain that piece of learning. In this regard, we should try to keep our comments brief and let the learner do most of the talking.

We should also avoid being repetitive because it is both time consuming and unnecessary. It appears to happen when insufficient clues are sent out to the critiquer that the pearls of wisdom have been received. This could be because of lack of understanding, because the cues are subtle, or because repetition has led to defensiveness. Ensure that the point has been understood then move on. The best way to do this is to use advocacy with inquiry.

Try also to avoid either making the other person defensive or becoming defensive yourself. If you detect that you have an abnormally strong response then question yourself and assume that the other person has a good reason for acting as they did. It is likely that they have hit one of your triggers and you are over-reacting as a result of previous learnt patterns of behaviour. Examples of actions that have led to unusually strong reactions include the following:

- Someone who is yawning or keeps fidgeting during a session.
- Mobile phones going off.
- A candidate constantly bringing their own personal experiences to the session.
- A very disorganised approach which impinges on other peoples' experience.

It is worthwhile to reflect on your triggers because by knowing what they are you are more likely to be able to measure your response.

When giving feedback we ask a lot of a learner and occasionally they are clearly not ready to be critiqued and to comment on their own performance immediately. This is where good facilitation involves a flexible approach, moving away from the formula. At this point, we can sometimes give the learner space by shifting the focus and asking the whole group what additional strategies they might employ in a similar situation. The group often comes up with ideas, which the instructor would not have thought of. This ensures that the whole group is part of the learning event, the learner does not feel victimised and the pressures of the situation, which are artificially high, are lessened (Box 8.10).

When you get to the stage in a critique where it is appropriate to make comments and suggestions for changes in behaviour make them relevant, specific, concrete and achievable.

- *Relevant*: Avoid commenting on aspects of a person's manner that are not relevant.

Box 8.10 Using the ideas of the group by posing a specific question

'When you asked the nurse to put on the monitors and take some bloods at the same time he got in your way and achieved neither of the tasks. What alternatives can anyone suggest for that difficult situation?'

Following the suggestions
'Which of those do you think that you would feel most comfortable saying/doing?'

- *Specific*: Use phrases such as *'When you did X'* rather than *'You have a tendency to…'*, thus use what you have observed (rather than inferred) to illustrate the point that you are making.
- *Concrete*: Make concrete suggestions for change, for example *'You need to assess the patient's GCS in order to fill out the triage form'*. This would be more helpful than *'Have a bit of a think about how you use the triage card'*.
- *Achievable*: Do not overwhelm the candidate by either giving too much feedback or suggesting outcomes that are not achievable within the time frame. It is often possible to make different teaching points from the two or three scenarios you run consecutively. Candidates sometimes learn as much from their peers' scenarios and critique as they do from their own because their stress levels are lower. Consequently you can measure out the feedback and learning points that you make over the course of the session (Box 8.11).

Box 8.11 Giving concrete, achievable feedback

'You were struggling with the drug dosages but that is something that you can easily find out. I suggest you read them up and learn them so that in your next practice, or when you are faced with this situation for real, you don't put yourself in a similar position of potentially making the situation worse. Would you be able to find time to do that?'

Summary and learning

Critiquing is one of the most valuable aspects of any teaching and learning environment where practical situations and role-plays are encountered. In order to critique well ensure that you maintain your credibility with the group, are honest and helpful in the feedback that you give and engage in an informed and relevant dialogue with the learner.

References

Luft J. *Group Processes: An Introduction to Group Dynamics*, 2nd edn. Mayfield, Palo Alto, 1979.

Maslow A. *Motivation and Personality*, 3rd edn. Harper & Row, New York, 1987.

Pendleton D, Schofield, T, Havelock, P & Tate P. *The Consultation: An Approach to Learning and Teaching*. Oxford University Press, Oxford, 1984.

CHAPTER 9

E-learning

Learning outcomes

By the end of this chapter you should be able to demonstrate an understanding of:
- The nature of the e-learning experience from the point of view of the learner and of the facilitator

Introduction

E-learning, or online learning, has had a surprisingly long history: it is over 40 years since computers first made their presence felt in higher education and over 10 years since dedicated computer platforms, subsequently called virtual learning environments (VLEs), first appeared. Funders of training across the world are beginning to suggest the emerging importance of e-learning. Sensing this philosophical shift, both ALSG and RC (UK) are adapting traditional resuscitation courses to look at mixed mode learning, combining the benefits of e-learning materials and traditional face-to-face teaching. Other contemporary developments within resuscitation are software simulations delivered through an e-learning platform.

Regardless of the particular software platform, VLEs share similar characteristics and in this chapter we will explore these from a number of perspectives.

Initially institutions (mis)used the internet by the wholesale transfer of face to face courses from the conventional classroom to the virtual classroom, without taking the change in pedagogy into account. The inevitable outcome of this is that the worst features of the conventional classroom (i.e. a non-interactive lecture)

Pocket Guide to Teaching for Medical Instructors, Second Edition. Edited by Ian Bullock, Mike Davis, Andrew Lockey and Kevin Mackway-Jones. © 2008 Blackwell Publishing, ISBN: 978-1-4051-7569-2.

are transplanted onto a computer screen. Thus the learner's role is translated from passive listening in a lecture theatre to passive reading at a computer.

This situation changed because of the influence of a number of educational technologists during the late 1990s. In more recent online environments learners are able to engage with materials in a more dynamic way through the use of a number of key characteristics:

- Text
- Tables
- Illustrations
- Hyperlinks to other websites, including audio and video clips, and other
- (reusable) learning objects
- Synchronous and asynchronous discussions.

Text

This is probably self-evident – except to say that online discourse has developed some of its own characteristics. This is a slightly more informal read and a more direct approach than (say) a text book. In addition to the main dialogue, text can also include hypertext links (hot links) to other text-based sites to demonstrate or amplify an argument. It may be useful to think of this as a dynamic referencing system.

Tables, graphs and other manifestations of data

These can either be drawn on the site, or links to documents can be provided.

Other hyperlinks

These can include websites, discussion areas, live feeds (e.g. RSS), podcasts and other audio and video feeds.

In some respects, all of the external links to the core text are what have come to be known as reusable learning objects. They are reusable in that they can be used in a wide variety of contexts, so have generic qualities and can also be accessed by any number of students in their original state. They range from simple matching, pairing and prioritising activities to more complex animated teaching and learning tasks involving the virtual entry into a simulated environment.

In addition to these animated sites, the use of video and audio clips can add to the richness and complexity of the material. As an example the medium of a videoed case conference or a disclosure interview in a child protection course can add considerably to the text.

Table 9.1 Forms of discussion

	Same time	Different time
Same place	Face to face meeting; synchronous conference	Asynchronous conference
Different place	Synchronous conference	Asynchronous conference

Discussion areas

Online discussions can be either synchronous or asynchronous. The key characteristics of these two forms are shown in Table 9.1.

The asynchronous conference has a place in the lives of busy people who find it difficult to make arrangements for face to face meetings, teleconferences or online, synchronous conferences. As will be evident from the table, face to face conversations are the least easy to populate but are considered by many to be a helpful component of an online course. This blended approach gives course organisers the opportunity to develop what experts in group dynamics call 'a good group', that is one that can function with a clear sense of purpose, secure boundaries, the ability to manage conflict and disagreement. This is particularly important and much harder to achieve online when participants find it difficult to sense who they are writing to.

There are a number of benefits and related challenges to working in a VLE and these are summarised in Table 9.2.

Table 9.2 Benefits and challenges to working in a VLE

Benefits	Challenges
Convenience of time and place means minimal disruption to family and work	Feelings of information overload and difficulty following the thread of the conversations
Fosters collaboration rather than competition	Increased time on task (for students and facilitators) and a tendency to access the site at all hours of the day
Allows for deeper critical thinking and reflection because of the time delay of asynchronous conferencing which in turn contributes to the building of ideas	Technical frustrations because of the steep learning curve for any new platform, access problems, password difficulties

Continued

Table 9.2 *Continued.*

Benefits	Challenges
The written record of the discussion aids the process of critical reflection	The written record sometimes inhibits learners who prefer the transitory nature of the spoken word: this is particularly true with discussions of a sensitive nature
Increased access to databases and a wealth of online resources	Potential for misunderstanding due to single cue (i.e. the words on the screen)
Students have ready access to a tutor or facilitator	Disjointed nature of conversation because of time delay
Cost effective because reduction in travel, hotels, time away from work	Students expect immediate responses from tutor
	The development costs can be high

Some of the challenges appear too difficult to overcome. Take, for example, skills teaching. Conventionally the preferred method of teaching skills is the four-stage approach – all four stages taking place in a single session. However, an online approach to skills teaching might consist of video clips of stages 1 and 2 followed by reinforcement and practice in a face to face session. An advantage of this would be that the video could include closeup shots of the skill, interspersed with clinical information or contexts, diagrams, photographs, etc. Furthermore, online learners can play the video as many times as they want (both before and after the face-to-face session).

VLEs can therefore supplement rather than replace face to face activity. Some aspects of face to face work cannot currently be easily replicated online – for example, role-play, scenarios and skills teaching. However, the VLE can be useful for the transference of knowledge-based content and for discussions about case studies. Knowledge based programmes, clinical case study programmes and diagnostic support systems provide current UK medical trainees with important access to material through e-learning. The introduction of the 'Foundation Programme' in 2005, for junior doctors, demonstrates the increasing interest in the role of e-learning to support both trainers and trainees.

What follows is an exploration of some of the issues associated with running the interactive elements of blended courses.

Facilitating online learning

Facilitating an online discussion is similar in certain ways to facilitating an open discussion. It is also very different and we will now go on to discuss how it is best done, giving examples from actual online discussions to illustrate.

There are some behaviours that encourage online learning and others that do not. Look at Table 9.3 and consider which column is likely to facilitate and which inhibits learning.

Table 9.3 Behaviours

Facing conflict	Pacifying
Building ideas	Working independently
Social activity	Lack of socialising
Risk taking	Closing down enquiry
Expressing interest	Lack of interest
Humour	Lack of humour
Reflecting	Ignoring the process
Feedback/Disclosure	Denial
Challenging	Unquestioning acceptance

As you can see, the left-hand column in Table 9.3 shows the behaviours that encourage and facilitate learning in both self and others, while the right-hand column shows behaviours that have the opposite effect. Part of the role of the facilitator is to recognise those behaviours and to prevent them from becoming norms – that is the tacit imperatives that can govern group behaviour.

These left-hand behaviours can be divided into 'group' and 'learning' dynamics. Some may belong to both, as shown in Table 9.4.

Table 9.4 Group and learning dynamics

Group dynamics	Learning dynamics
Risk taking	Building ideas
Facing conflict	Challenging
Social activity	Experimenting
Humour	Metacommunication
Reflecting on the process	Reflecting on the process
Feedback/Disclosure	Feedback/Disclosure
Expressing interest	

Davis and Denning (2001) have demonstrated the relationship between the two in a 2 × 2 matrix shown in Figure 9.1.

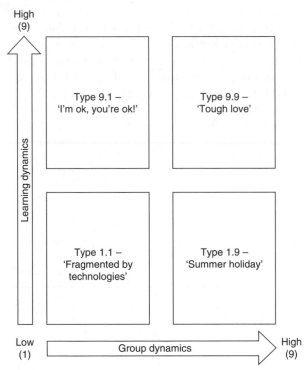

Figure 9.1 Group and learning dynamics.

Web conference

A conference works best if it is functioning in 'tough love' mode and what follows will describe some of its characteristics, including:

- Authenticity
- Shared ownership
- Creativity
- Interdependence
- Autonomy
- Exchange of social capital

Each of these will be considered in turn.

Authenticity

As in all conversations, there would be better outcomes if people said what they meant, rather than trying to dress it up to make them or their listeners more comfortable. This, however, is easier said than done. It may be best to think of what kinds of things to avoid:

- Generalisation – *'Thank you for your excellent contribution'*
- Vagueness – *'What you write is very interesting ...'*
- False consensus – *'I am sure we all agree that ...'*

The most authentic interventions are those that are grounded in reality: in other words, people say what they mean and use evidence from what was actually written together with their reasoning to support their positions.

Jeremy: 'The definition of discipline you quote makes me a little uneasy'.

Shared ownership

Shared ownership is of the experience and the conclusions (however tentative) that can be drawn from them. Learners will have had a range of experiences and have access to bodies of knowledge that they can offer to the group. In the early days of a conference the learners often make isolated comments, but they usually begin to use each others' thoughts to spark their own after a while. Some people are particularly adept at this and are referred to as 'virtuosos'. Those who have a facility for online communication are not necessarily those who are active group members in a face to face situation. In fact it is often people who have a slower, more reflective approach, which can deny them the opportunity to talk face to face, who in fact blossom online. An asynchronous learning space is potentially a thoughtful, creative, challenging place.

Norah: 'Anyway, after reading Kate's last contribution I decided to check the dictionary for the definition of discipline'.

The role of the facilitator is to enable this process. An over-dominant facilitator who is keen to share knowledge and experience can disrupt this process for the learners, and this trait should be avoided.

Creativity

Groups can often come to highly creative solutions – particularly when there is no right answer.

Maureen: 'I have been reading all the thoughtful responses to your question, Josie, and am very worried that I never considered this as a possibility!'

This outcome rarely emerges from an over-facilitated session since the group may spend too much time looking for the 'correct' solution or attempting to please the facilitator.

Autonomy

If the group members are self-determining and are functioning as adults they will have autonomy. In order to give students the space to express their autonomy it is the facilitator's role to ask challenging questions. In order to facilitate deeper learning consider a range of questions such as the following:

- To answer this question, what other questions must we answer first?
- What is an alternative?
- How could we find out if that was so?
- How does that apply to this case?
- Could you explain your reasoning on this?
- What assumptions are being made here?
- In order to help me understand better, could you give an example of that?
- When you wrote 'X' I understood you to mean 'Y', is that what you intended?
- I am not quite clear what you mean by 'X'.

Even before this can happen, though, students need to feel that their attempts within the conference are valued and the first days of a conference can be extremely nerve-wracking for a facilitator as very few students respond to prompts. Some learners lack confidence and need to be encouraged, sometimes by email, sometimes even by phone initially. As soon as students begin to respond to each other the facilitator can lessen their involvement whilst continuing to observe. It becomes important to monitor without responding: when students pose questions, wait, and then wait again for someone else to reply.

Exchange of social capital

An important element if people are to be able to take risks and offer challenges is the social dimension to interaction which is often taken for granted face to face. It happens before, after and during lessons and is often effortlessly incorporated into the learning. As with other aspects of the VLE it needs to be a little more self-conscious online and can be encouraged in online ice-breaking sessions, in the creation of a café area for social chat or through deliberately making brief off-task comments.

As in face to face groups, online groups quickly develop a language of their own and in-jokes. These are important to the cohesion of the group whilst they might appear to detract from the learning. Standard jokes do not always work online as they are often contingent on timing and pace. Humour which arises out of knowledge of each other is more likely to be successful.

> *Sally-Anne*: 'Mike what sort of time is that to be up at the computer have you got jet lag?! Or did the rain wake you?'

Interdependence

This is probably the main characteristic of 'tough love'. The group have high expectations of one another and expect all of the above features to be manifested in their exchanges.

> *Maureen*: 'It really has been great 'chatting' on these e-discussions – I have learnt a lot in the process. Haven't we been lucky to have a group which has worked well together?'

At this point, the role of the facilitator is to stand back. They may occasionally have to summarise and redirect but not to evaluate.

Summary and learning

E-learning has been around for some time, but has only recently been transformed into the active learning environment required by adult learners. Instructors facilitating online learning need to ensure they understand the basic attributes of the e-learning environment. Once they have done this they can begin to facilitate and manage e-learners.

Reference

Davis M & Denning K. Almost as helpful as good theory: some conceptual possibilities for the online classroom. *Association for Learning Technology Journal* 2001; **9**(2): 64–75.

CHAPTER 10
The role of the instructor

Learning outcomes

By the end of this chapter you should be able to demonstrate an understanding of:
- The prerequisites for instructor status
- The essential qualities of an instructor
- Mentoring

Introduction

There are a number of reasons why individuals become instructors. It may be because they enjoy teaching or because they are actively involved in a specialty or job that has a teaching commitment. It may be that becoming an instructor is an integral part of their career plan. Whatever the reasons, the role is both rewarding and motivating. Most instructors find that combining the theory learnt on courses with practical experience helps to increase or maintain their own motivation. Finally, many find that although the role of an instructor is demanding and there are no financial rewards, it is an enjoyable, sociable and worthwhile activity.

What makes a good instructor?

Good instructors have a strong foundation of knowledge and skill that allow them to become (or at least aspire to becoming) role models for learners. The building blocks for this have been described by Hesketh et al (2001) and are shown in Figure 10.1.

Pocket Guide to Teaching for Medical Instructors, Second Edition. Edited by Ian Bullock, Mike Davis, Andrew Lockey and Kevin Mackway-Jones. © 2008 Blackwell Publishing, ISBN: 978-1-4051-7569-2.

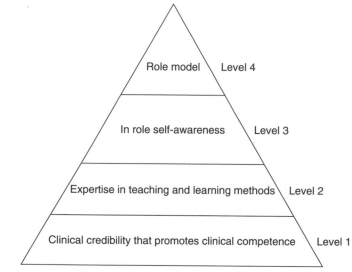

Figure 10.1   Building blocks of an instructor.

Level 1: clinical credibility

The foundations for instructor performance are the knowledge, skills and experience that each individual brings to their role. This means that ability to teach includes an ability to demonstrate:

- Clinical application of the theoretical content from the provider course;
- Understanding of the clinical context;
- Knowledge and credibility.

Level 2: expertise in teaching and learning methods

A good instructor will make learning relevant, meaningful and fun, with all teaching sessions prepared thoroughly. Contrary to traditional approaches in healthcare and medical education, candidates will not simply consume what is read and said to them. Teaching is about providing the optimal conditions for effective learning, where candidates become active participants in the learning process. Key components for instructors to be able to achieve this are competency in teaching methods and understanding of how to facilitate candidate learning.

Level 3: in role self-awareness

A good instructor, by being aware of themselves and the learners' needs and abilities, adds a dynamic quality to the learning experience so that more than simple content is being covered. A key attribute is the ability to recognise the individual needs and strengths of each candidate. Understanding the principles outlined in this book, combined with good interpersonal skills and a healthy attitude in the learning environment, should enable the instructor to provide feedback and support, enabling candidate growth and development.

Level 4: role model

Experienced instructors will tell you that they themselves learn something new from each course they attend. Their ability to reflect and learn in action (on the job) adds to their credibility as an instructor. Remember, Learning is a journey not a destination. Capturing this journey is encouraged and this can be achieved by maintaining a professional portfolio, where experiences gained can be maximised through reflection on practice.

Mentorship

Most courses require instructors to act as mentors to specific groups of candidates. The role of the mentor is not always well defined and there is a wide variance in the practice of mentorship between instructors. There is little research that provides evidence as to a best practice model for mentorship. However, the principles of mentorship are widely published and a model may be constructed.

Mentorship can be defined as a relationship that fosters support in many areas including teaching, supervision, guidance, counselling, assessment and evaluation. It is clear that the instructor must remain focused on the outcomes required from mentor/mentee meetings and the following guidance may be of help. The mentor meetings should be structured in such a way as to give time for group mentorship as well as the all-important individual mentorship. It is vital that candidates are given the opportunity to discuss their individual needs away from the group and that this is seen as being a programmed element and not only reserved for the struggling candidate.

The key role of the mentor is as teacher and critical friend. The teacher element is less distinct during time-limited mentor/mentee meetings. Mentors should be aware of who their specific group is and observe their development throughout the course, giving structured feedback when and where appropriate. This naturally leads to the critical friend role whereby mentors can give open and honest feedback having developed a level of rapport with their mentees.

The model in Box 10.1 may prove useful in structuring a 15-minute mentor meeting and follows the principles of feedback already discussed in Chapter 8. However, it is also important to remember the value of a more flexible approach, which will appeal to some learners.

Box 10.1 Suggested guidance for mentor meetings

Guidance for conduct of short mentor/mentee meetings
9 minutes – group critique
1 Engage group and ask them to critique course so far.
2 Critique group including their teamwork and address any issues with group dynamics exploring strategies for improvement.
3 *Pragmatics*: Run through any course administration required by course director. Confirm next start time. Close group and explain all will receive individual feedback.

6 minutes total – individual feedback (2 minutes for all candidates if instructors paired up for mentorship)
4 *Individual feedback*: Discuss any strategies that may help improve individual performance and give clear take home message if necessary. If doing well, a clear message is also required. Close with candidate and invite next person.

Initial mentor meetings may not be very productive especially if the mentors have had little contact with their mentees. This is where instructor responsibilities as a mentor become clear. The instructor who 'has to leave early' or is late in arriving to the course will not be in a position to offer professional mentorship and risks losing credibility from the point of view of the mentees. A good course timetable will arrange for mentors to be grouped together having contact with their mentees at the beginning and end of day 1 and during the skill station rotations, allowing for much more objective mentoring. In addition, important information about a candidate's performance may only become evident at the faculty meeting, after the course has dispersed for the day. Mentors must ensure that they feedback any relevant information to their mentees before commencement of the following day's course.

Attending meetings

On many organised courses there are faculty meetings at the beginning of the course and at the end of each day. The initial meeting is a forum for all instructors to meet since often they may not know each other and have probably not all taught together before. The course director and the course co-ordinator can introduce instructors to each other, discuss the layout of the teaching environment, note any last minute changes to the programme and importantly, discuss the approach to any contentious areas that are being addressed.

The initial meeting also provides an opportunity to ensure that all instructors are prepared for the day ahead. Instructors teaching overlapping topics can use the opportunity to check which areas they are each covering and to ensure a consistent approach.

Faculty meetings at the end of the day should be more focused on the candidates themselves, although any logistical or controversial issues, which have arisen during the day may be discussed and rectified. The main aim of the discussion about the candidates is to identify those who need remedial help and to formulate a plan to deliver this. The assessments, which are collated from any formative feedback sheets should be used to assist in this process.

At the final faculty meeting, any formative and summative assessments are discussed. On some courses, learners may pass, retest in a particular area or it may be recommended that they repeat the course in its entirety. Some participants may be offered the opportunity to teach.

Supporting other instructors

Occasionally, the instructor who is carrying out a session is less confident and may require both moral and actual support. Instructors must show support for instructors in this position both by being there (for instance, by sitting in at the back of the lecture room) and by stepping in to answer difficult questions raised by candidates.

Regulations and requirements

Each governing body has similar, but slightly differing regulations with regard to completing instructor candidacies, maintaining instructor status, recertification and a code of conduct, it is important to familiarise yourself with these early on.

Many governing bodies maintain central lists of all qualified instructors and these are made available to course centres to allow them to invite instructors. Instructors will also be sent lists of the course centres and course dates to allow them to approach suitable centres if they so wish.

Summary and learning

As an instructor, you will be part of a faculty of experienced people teaching knowledge and skills to adult learners. The instructor role is rewarding and demands highly motivated and reliable individuals who display knowledge and credibility in the field of resuscitation.

References

Hesketh E, Bagnall G, Buckley E, Friedman M, Goodall M, Harden R, Laidlaw J, Leighton-Beck L, McKinley P, Newton R & Oughton R. A framework for developing excellence as a clinical educator. *Medical Education* 2001; **35**(6): 555–564.

CHAPTER 11
Annotated bibliography

Boud D, Cohen R & Walker D, eds. *Using Experience for Learning.* SRHE and Open University Press, Buckingham, 1993.
[One of many collaborations with Boud on the contribution of reflection to adult learning in higher education and professional practice.]

Brookfield S. *Becoming a Critically Reflective Teacher.* Jossey-Bass, San Francisco, 1995.
[This is a powerful account of some of the social–psychological issues associated with being a teacher.]

Dewey J. *How We Think. A Restatement of the Relation of Reflective Thinking to the Educative Process*, Revised edn. D. C. Heath, Boston, 1933.
[Dewey laid the foundations for explorations of the significance of collaborative learning; the nature and potential of experience; and reflective practice. His books made a significant contribution to the thinking of authors like David Boud (*Reflection*), David Kolb (*Learning from Experience*) and Schön (*The Reflective Practitioner*). A new edition of this work was published in 2007.]

Knowles MS. *The Adult Learner. A Neglected Species*, 4th edn. Gulf Publishing, Houston, 1990.
[A seminal work in adult learning surveys adult learning theories and explores further his notion of andragogy which has been described as 'the art of helping adults learn' as opposed to pedagogy, 'the science or art of teaching'.]

Kolb D. *Experiential Learning: Experiences as the Source of Learning and Development.* Prentice-Hall, Englewood Cliffs, 1984.

Pocket Guide to Teaching for Medical Instructors, Second Edition. Edited by Ian Bullock, Mike Davis, Andrew Lockey and Kevin Mackway-Jones. © 2008 Blackwell Publishing, ISBN: 978-1-4051-7569-2.

[An exploration of the significance of learning from experience and what is required to develop the capacity to do so. Further work with Fry (Kolb D & Fry R. 'Toward an applied theory of experiential learning'. In: Cooper C, ed. *Theories of Group Process*, John Wiley, London, 1975) created the learning styles inventory.

While aspects of Kolb's work have been criticised for apparent inattention to some detail, it still makes a valuable contribution to understanding of what is required if we are to learn from experience.]

Lewin K. *Field Theory in Social Science: Selected Theoretical Papers.* In: Cartwright D, ed. Harper & Row, New York, 1951.

[Almost all of Kurt Lewin's publications appeared after his death in editions edited by his graduate students, many of whom became major contributors to our understanding of adult learning, particularly in groups. He is also credited with creating the idea of 'action research', described as:

a form of self-reflective enquiry undertaken by participants in social situations in order to improve the rationality and justice of their own practices, their understanding of these practices, and the situations in which the practices are carried out

Carr W & Kemmis S. Becoming Critical. Education,
Knowledge and Action Research, Falmer, Lewes.

More recent collection of Lewin's work can be found at Gold M. *The Complete Social Scientist.* APA Books, Washington, 1999.]

Maslow A. A theory of human motivation. *Psychological Review* 1943; **50**: 370–396.

[This article has been a major contributor to thinking about motivation and how that impacts on learning.]

Schön D. *The Reflective Practitioner: How Professionals Think in Action.* Basic Books, New York, 1983.

[Among Schön's concerns was that university education did not necessarily relate to the day to day practices of the expert practitioner. Schön's target behaviour for professionals is the capacity to reflect-in-action, rather than reflect-on-action. However, the capacity to engage in the latter may be a prerequisite of the former.]

Index